CANDIDA, the epidemic of this century: SOLVED

LUC DE SCHEPPER
M.D. PH.D. C.A.

l.d.s. publications
4318 beaucroft ct.
westlake village, ca. 91361

Acknowledgments

All my patients have contributed to this work, through their questions, their concerns and positive attitudes. Some of them have stood out, either through their direct contribution, such as my dear friends Mark Fowler and Gloria Axelrod, or through their insight and intelligent questions, such as Bonnie Armstrong, Phil Gernhard, Joan Hayes, Maria Grimm, Geraldine Boyd, Diane Raiskin, Lynn Schermerhorn, Kaj Lohman, Carol Vogelman, Nancy Knupfer, Marjorie Buetell, Jan Carter, Candice Goodfellow, and many more.

Anyone afflicted by this disease should consult a nutritional, holistic-oriented doctor. This book is not intended to be used as a self-therapy guide but, hopefully, will give some more insight, hope and return to a better health and fulfilling life.

Dr. Luc De Schepper
2901 Wilshire Boulevard
Suite 435
Santa Monica, CA   90403
(213) 828-4480

Table of Contents

1
Profile of a Killer Disease

Egypt, 1924: British egyptologist, Hugh Evelyn-White, was among the first to enter the tomb of King Tutankhamen, shortly after its discovery in 1922 near the ruins of Luxor. Evelyn-White became one of the dozen explorers to die soon after visiting the site. "I have succumbed to a curse," wrote he in his own blood in 1924, moments before hanging himself. At the time no one could explain his suicide nor the many other mysterious deaths of other unfortunate ones who had entered the tomb. Coming primarily to look for gold and treasures, the excavators paid no attention to the pink, gray and green patches of fungi on the chamber walls. So, in reality, King Tut's curse was a really severe allergic reaction to fungi: fruits and vegetables placed in the tomb to feed the pharaoh throughout eternity but which, decaying over centuries, had created deadly molds.

U.S.A., 1985: Headlines state that a certain killer-disease has claimed the lives of five infants in a local Los Angeles hospital, while another fourteen suffering from the same problems survived. The cause of the deaths was respiratory infections, complicated by yeast infections. The children were as young as six months of age. Yet those infants could only breathe with the assistance of plastic tubes inserted into their tracheas. The yeast-organism was found to be present in the tracheas of each of the infants, while in fifty-percent of the cases, the yeast was discovered in the blood and urine in the dead babies.

U.S.A., 1985: A 20-year old girl is in a car accident causing her severe head trauma, missing and broken teeth, multiple sprains and strains to the neck, arms and legs. Physical therapy and major dental restorative surgery, under the coverage of heavy antibiotic therapy were routine measures taken in the hospital. However, two months later, she experienced a series of symptoms, getting gradually worse: increasing fatigue, feeling of spaciness, ravenous appetite and rapid weight gain. Later, she experienced attacks that were diagnosed by neurologists as complex partial seizures (drowsiness, fatigue, confusion, anxiety, crying, loss of perception and, eventually, shock). Duration and intensity varied from attack to attack. On numerous occasions she was taken to the emergency room, diagnosed as a mental case, and released without further treatment. Before coming to my office, she was confused and considered herself a hypochondriac, since she had been treated as such by most doctors. Miraculously, she was free of 'seizures' after a course of anti-yeast medication, a change of diet, and a move away from the smoggy Los Angeles area to the clearer air of the mountains.

USA, June '86: headlines in the L.A. Times: "Chronic Flu-like Illness, a medical Mystery Story." S. Smith, 42, came down with the mysterious illness soon after she ran a marathon in San Francisco last year. She got better before becoming sick again this spring, forcing her to quit her job as a business manager. Running even a half mile now would "put me in bed for a day and a half", she said. Smith is among 160 residents of Lake Tahoe's North Shore who have been diagnosed by two local physicians since the winter of 1985 as having a chronic flu-like illness in a medical puzzle that has assumed national proportions. Most of the victims are well-educated, previously healthy, more likely to be women than men and about 40 years old (the "baby boomers!"). Their complaints also are similar: severe fatigue, recurrent colds and difficulties with memory and concentration. About half of them have enlarged lymph nodes in their neck and almost all of them have abnormal blood tests, suggesting that a common viral infection may be involved: the EBV or Ebstein Barr Virus. The best the two local doctors could come up with was a diagnosis, "a chronic version of the more familiar Ebstein Barr virus." "Many of the patients had first seen other physicians who either "didn't know what was going on or thought the patients were crazy." One victim recalled: "My days are pretty boring. I read or get a videocassette. I feel like a Raggedy Ann with no stuffing." In their serial of patients, about 50% are as ill today as when they were first diagnosed, about 25% have waxing and waning symptoms, and about 25% feel they have recovered. Another doctor concluded: "He had seen several hundred patients who he believes have the disease. The illness exists. There is a very clear picture. The patients can't go to work or school. Their marriages break up. All aspects of life are interfered with."

Do all these stories harking back almost a century have anything in common? Yes, they do! No matter how different these stories may sound, they all involve yeast infections.

Finally, a particularly frightening and sad story reached me from another State. The girl is fifteen years old by now, but she had been suffering from colic since birth. In addition, she was plagued with continuous colds which she fought with an average of at least twelve courses of anti-biotics per year. And this, for the first six years of her life. Life was never normal for this poor patient. She felt tightness in the chest, dizziness, depression, a sense of inner frailty or shakiness; she had headaches, difficulty breathing and was also observed to have numerous airborne and food allergies. The school environment made her deathly ill;

numerous consultations with doctors had disastrous consequences. Finally, the family moved from California to Texas, to the "world's expert help center for environmental illnesses." Aside from draining the family coffers and further deteriorating the patient's health, nothing was accomplished. The family finally moved to Colorado and rented an ecology house (in the middle of the woods, no roads, no gas stove, no carpets, etc.).

The mother, desperate with the minimal help she received from health professionals, decided to take matters in her own hands. Rotation diet, daily exercise, vitamins and minerals, massage, touch therapy and laugh therapy brought her daughter back to a healthier status, but she still cannot leave the house at all. Weakness of limbs is still a problem; food intake has to be monitored carefully.

WHAT IS CANDIDA ALBICANS?

This infamous yeast or fungus does not manufacture its own food from the sun as plants do, but rather consumes it like animals, burning fuel foods with oxygen. These tiny microflora are everywhere, subsisting on the surface of all living things. These are the yeasts that cause the bread to rise and fruit to ferment into wine. Normally, this candida is always present on the internal and external body surfaces (skin, mucosae and digestive tract). It is especially present in the esophagus (causing a symptom such as "food sticking in the throat with impossibility of swallowing") and in the small intestine. Normally, these yeast cells live in harmony with other bacteria in a concentration of millions of bacteria versus one candida. These bacteria form the normal flora of the gastro-intestinal tract and inhibit the overgrowth of yeast in normal circumstances.

WHY IS THIS DISEASE SHOWING UP IN EPIDEMIC PROPORTIONS?

Historically, we know, of course, that candidiasis has been around for centuries. Both oral and vaginal trush were in existence over two thousand years ago. And, if we accept that scientists working prior to 1980 were good at what they did, it seems unlikely that they would have been unaware of what a dreadful disease Candida was. I believe there is another reason for this: widespread Candida is a <u>new</u> problem. We are currently witnessing a virtual epidemic of Candidiasis. Only a few years ago, yeast diseases were called in the medical world, the diseases of the future. The doctor reviewing the recent literature will conclude that the future is now <u>here</u>!

2

Causes

What have we changed in the recent decades that we have created such an opportune milieu for these yeast bugs?

Any cause of disease can be reduced to four main groups: **HEREDITARY FACTORS - FOOD - EMOTIONS and EXTERNAL FACTORS.**

For certain diseases, the cause will overwhelmingly be one of these four, but usually all of them are involved to a certain degree. The ONE group of factors, however, that predominates in the outbreak of Candida is the external group.

When our first antibiotics were made available during the Second World War (Penicillin), indisputably we had made a big step forward, but things got somewhat out-of-hand after that initial period. Broad spectrum antibiotics were--and are-- used for common colds so that the normal flora (coli, bacteroides and enterobacterias) can be suppressed. We all know of the use of tetracyclines in the therapy for acne; low doses were, and still are, given for months at a time. Ampicillin and Bactrim are frequently given for the wrong reasons, or by request from a public that insists on strong medication for a cold since they have no time [since life's constraints do not allow the time for a natural healing] to heal more naturally. The "time is money" attitude which dictates this behavior is not necessarily the wisest approach, as we are now discovering.

A lot of my patients tell me that the routine adding of antibiotics to the feed of chickens, cows and pigs is driving them to vegetarianism. This is not an unusual reaction. Many see little good in this practice and the potential for harm. Although people who raise cows or pigs insist that they must use antibiotics to prevent infections and promote growth, knowledgeable critics are now blowing the whistle on them and raise the red flag.

Authorities in England put a stop to adding low doses of antibiotics to the feed of livestock and poultry in 1971. So did a number of other countries in Europe. The FDA recommended a similar ban in 1977. However, Congress said "no," proposing that more data was needed to make certain that tetracycline added to the animal food posed a serious threat to the nation's health.

The gravest threat is that regular feeding of antibiotics may produce bacteria resistant to it, and lead to their multiplication in the flesh of the animal. The problem gets worse when people ingest antibiotics, thus killing off their healthy intestinal bacteria and allowing the overgrowth of yeast cells.

Only two days of antibiotics allows the overgrowth of Candida in a susceptible patient. And, although antibiotics may be the main culprits, they are not the only ones! Cytostatica, immunosuppressives and cortisone are the cornerstones of many cancer therapies. These forms of therapy decrease the activity of the "liver filter." The liver, the largest gland in the body, has many functions. These include the formation of bile, carbohydrate storage, ketone body formation and other functions in the control of carbohydrate metabolism. Other functions include the detoxification of many drugs and toxins, manufacturing of many plasma proteins, urea formation and many important functions in the fat metabolism.

Other exterior factors are surgical interventions, burns,

catheterizations, dialysis, diabetes mellitus, hypothyroidism, hormonal therapy ("the pill"), pregnancy and a ferriprive anemia.   All patients in this group have an increased
risk for yeast infections.

The other three factor groups, hereditary - food-
emotions, are by no means to be neglected in favoring an
outbreak of Candida.

Hereditary factors are important in a way and we cannot
change them, of course, but we must be aware of the potential
dangers we run if we neglect to protect ourselves.   How many
times will patients recognize that their parents went through
the same symptom complex, and accepted it like victims since
clear diagnosis was impossible back then.   If a person knows
he risks a certain disease since the incidence is high in the
family history, taking the three other factors -- food,
emotions and external -- into account, will help him avoid
that same disease.

Food plays an extremely important role in the outbreak of
Candida.   Yeast-containing foods are everywhere in our diet
and we accentuate yeast growth by the way we process foods.
More about the diet aspect is discussed in the therapy
section.

Perhaps the least considered factor is emotional. Emotions
are part of the pathogenesis of every disease; this is more
and more recognized.   In the case of yeast infection, it is
generated by worry and obsession that gradually lead to an
attenuated immune system.   Patients affected by Candidiasis
are mostly worriers, highly analytical, calculating, per-
fectionistic persons, with a tendency to keep their feelings
inward.   More about the emotions is found in Chapter #7, "The
Psychological Profile of the Candida Patient."

3

Symptoms of Candida Infections

So, how do we recognize that we may possibly be a yeast patient, or in other words, what is the typical profile of a Candida patient?

The symptomatology of Candidiasis is a doctor's delight! Don't misunderstand me. It is not because the diagnosis is easy, but the broad pattern of symptoms gives each specialist in the medical field the opportunity to have a crack at this disease. That is exactly what happens. Patients consult their gynecologists for vaginal yeast infection and are prescribed anti-fungal cream or vaginal tablets to take as a result. The vaginal discharge seems to disappear after 5-6 days but recurs with the next menstrual cycle or right after sexual intercourse. Again, the same or maybe another local medication is prescribed. For women with the problem during intercourse, a low dosage is advised each time after intercourse. It is not fun anymore when this repeats itself over several years, and I am sure some people could even get tired of sex when it must be followed by yet another "pill."

At some point in the story, either the gynecologist or the patient gets tired of the situation and the focus will be shifted away to some other symptoms. There is a wide variety of choices here! Would we like to start with the allergic symptoms and spend a couple of thousand dollars on all the different food tests which inevitably will show some positive result? With the amount of preservatives, hormones and antibiotics we put in our food, it takes a very robust immune system not to crumble under the pressure. At this point, we go through our first change of diet. Swiftly, we omit some ten or twenty foods in our diet with oscillating results. We feel somewhat well on some days, but a lot worse on some other days. But do not become desperate. Another allergic test a couple of months later, shows some new food allergies! Again, twenty more foods are omitted from our diet and we start having problems to getting our daily menu together. And not rarely, it becomes impossible to eat at all, because we react on any food intake. "I am allergic to everything" and "I feel the best when I do not eat" are frequent complaints heard from such patients. Thirty pounds and two thousand dollars lighter, we finally find our way to the gastroenterologist because the bloating, gas and constipation becomes just too much for the patient (and his/her partner) to take. Upper and lower GI's are often taken and usually show nothing at all but an "irritable bowel syndrome" or "spastic colon." At this point, if we are lucky, some dietary advice is provided, but more likely, an anti-gas medication, laxative or anti-spasmodicum is prescribed. What a disappointment for patient and doctor when the symptoms have a tendency to aggravate. The thought that the symptoms might have something to do with our "nerves" is thrown into the air. That suggestion may prompt our psyche to go on with our quest for the healer. I am sure most Candida patients will see the ENT specialist for postnasal drip, the arthritis specialist for their muscle and joint pains, the urologist for their urinary symptoms, but the final specialist will, inevitably, be the psychiatrist!

Different specialists, fed up with the lack of results and the growing frustration of the patient, choose for the obvious cause: "It is all in your head" or "You have a psycho-somatic disease," is heard all over. Even the spouses at this moment are convinced that their partners either enjoy being sick or might have, indeed, something wrong emotionally.

Several visits to the emergency rooms for attacks, diagnosed as "hysteria," "hypoglycemia attacks" or "seizures" are only supporting the belief of the different doctors. Spouses accept it and what can the patient do at this point? Psychiatry seems to be the inevitable answer! Are we not suffering from mood swings, deep depressions, even suicidal tendencies? Memory and thinking seem to go up and down, while attention span has totally disappeared. I remember a patient who was a dance instructor. Standing in front of her class, she wanted to say: "Take your ankle," but she actually could not recall the word. Imagine the situation: 25 students staring at their teacher who is pointing at her ankle but cannot remember that simple word. No, it is no wonder, that almost ALL Candida patients land on the couch of the psychiatrist. Most of the attention at this point, of course, will be directed towards the depression which is severe in most cases. Rejection by everyone turned to, isolation in the family and loss of most friends, only add to the depression at this stage. And it becomes a long and expensive calvary: admission in a mental ward for some months and electro shocks would seem a logical step in the treatment. I can only feel great pity for Candida patients at this stage. Cut away from any support and subjected to hospital meals, they will get the final push. I wonder how many depressed patients we could find in those mental institutions that actually are Candida patients? We probably will never know.

In many publications you can read about medical breakthroughs and claims of discoveries of Candida or other yeast infections. However, as in many other areas of life, we have simply been blind to the factors of Candidiasis for a very long time.

Concerning Candida, all we have to do is look backwards to ancient medicines. Taking another approach allows an almost immediate diagnosis. However, not necessarily by the same name, but the name of a diagnosis has never guaranteed a good treatment. Let me prove it to you in the case of Candida. Already five thousand years ago, a Candida patient would have been diagnosed as having an "ENERGY-DEFICIENT SPLEEN-PANCREAS." (In Chinese medicine, both organs are considered as one.)

What are the functions of the spleen? The main function of this organ is transportation and transformation of food stuffs. It is the main organ of digestion and its proper function provides good appetite and good bowel movement. Lack of energy in this organ will, therefore, show initial gastrointestinal symptoms: bloating, abdominal distension, diarrhea changing quickly into constipation, loss of weight, although initially there might be a difficulty in losing weight, heartburn, indigestion, bad breath and mucus in the stools. Some foods such as raw and cold ones will decrease the energy in the spleen sooner than others, but when the deficiency becomes profound, any food intake will be followed by a reaction resembling an allergic symptom to those foods. In reality, they are not; it is the spleen showing it does not have the strength to do its job.

Another major function of the spleen is the production of the blood and, especially, white blood cells. Hence, its enormous importance in maintaining the immune system since white blood cells (T cells, B cells and Helper cells) are the defenders of our body. Deficient function will impair host deficiencies resulting in recurrent infections.

When we look at the prevalence of the modern diseases such as Ebstein Barr Virus (EBV), Cytomegaly Virus (CMV), re-current Herpes Simplex and AIDS, most of these diseases have many symptoms in common because all of them are spleen-deficient syndromes. Since the spleen is the blood producer for all the organs, a spleen deficiency translates into mental fatigue, drowsiness, inability to concentrate, dizziness, a drained feeling, a feeling of spaciness, poor memory and general numbness. These are all blood-deficiency symptoms.

According to acupuncture, the spleen not only produces the blood, but it is also responsible for keeping it in the vessels. Therefore, abnormal gum bleeding and menstrual irregularities, such as intermenstrual bleeding, polymenor-rhea, heavy bleeding and also, the other hormonal imbalances (PMS and Dysmenorrhea) may come into the picture.

The role of the spleen in our water metabolism is manifest at different levels: at that of the intestines --causing diarrhea--, at that of the bladder --causing anuria-- and at that of the subcutaneous level, producing edema.

There are some other interesting observations to be made on Candida patients and which are easily explained through acupuncture. Every Candida patient knows that s/he will be worse on muggy, damp days, or in houses with a lot of humidity and molds. There is also a typical craving for sweets. Five thousand years ago, the Chinese observed that there was a relationship between certain organs and climate factors (they called them the Exterior Pernicious factors). Cold was associated with the kidney organ, Heat with the heart, Dryness with the lung, Wind with the liver, and Dampness with the spleen. Humidity is THE enemy of the spleen, decreasing the energy in this organ dramatically. In the case of Candida, deficiency of Energy in the spleen is precisely the root of the problem.

Another relation exists between the organ and the tastes. To each organ belongs a taste which feeds the organic energy-deficiency if given in moderate quantities, but will decrease that same energy if consumed in high quantity. And we can guess it: the taste belonging to the spleen is sweet. Cravings for sweets are the major sign of a spleen in distress. Nutrasweet, for instance, which is supposedly five times sweeter than sugar, presents an increased danger for this organ.

And, is it not interesting that many Candida patients have been diagnosed as hypoglycemics? Remember what we said about the spleen-pancreas entity? In other words, hypoglycemia is nothing else than a precursor of the Candida. It makes such patient more susceptible to yeast infections. As we can see, patients with this syndrome were diagnosed 5000 years ago.

Another frequent symptom noted in the history of almost every Candida patient is "Cystitis": frequent urination, burning feeling and urgency. However, it is a big mistake frequently done by the patient and the medical profession to prescribe antibiotics BEFORE the result of the urine analysis AND culture, with sensitivity, has come back. Very frequently, the result will be negative since the elimination of the Candida via the urine will mimic these symptoms. Imagine the mistake done by giving antibiotics such as Bactrim and Ampicillin, frequently prescribed in these conditions. If you suffer from cystitis, you can always take cranberry juice (a natural killer of urinary bacterias) and Pyridium 200 mg, for the burning feeling. Once the results of the culture are known, if an antibiotic is necessary, at least you have the choice of the least damaging one. And, you can take the double doses of Acidophilus to protect the gastro-intestinal flora so that yeast infections are restricted to a minimum.

Another almost constant observation is the aggravation of symptoms one week before the menstrual cycle. Another possibility is the appearance of a vaginal infection just before the cycle. How can this be explained? The progesterone level increases the week before the bleeding. One of the effects of the increased progesterone is the increase of the glycemia (glucose in the blood). And, the sugar or glucose is exactly what those yeast cells thrive on. Inevitably in this period, the yeast infection which was latent in that patient, exacerbates and becomes clinical apparent. And, no wonder that cravings for sugar are most prominent at this moment: the increased amount of yeast cells wants food, they are, in fact, screaming for food and most patients oblige. Many patients with PMS will fall into this category: the increased sugar intake will make them depressive, irritable and subject to mood swings. As we can see with those patients, neither hormonal intake nor intake of the famous vitamin, B6, will improve this situation. One fact is sure: females with Candidiasis have PMS.

Another very annoying symptom is the irritation and burning feeling of all the mucosae: around the anus, the vagina, the mouth and lips, and even the mucosae of the stomach, which will create a constant hungry feeling. Again, knowledge of Acupuncture will save us here: the mucosae fall under the domain of the spleen; this organ is attacked by "Heat - Dampness." Frequently, the patient feels hot inside of his body. He can easily follow this up by looking at his tongue picture, especially in the morning: a thick yellow coating in the middle of the tongue is seen. When the patient gets better, the yellow thick coating becomes thin and whitish, the most objective sign s/he can observe.

A very annoying symptom is brainfog: concentration and attention span are minimal. It seems that a Candida patient has to read everything at least three times more than anybody else, and to his/her despair, s/he is unable to retain it. It also seems to be the symptom that disappears last: most of the symptoms have improved or disappeared before "the curtain lifts from their brain."

What are the causes? I think they are threefold. The first one is the formation of toxins, discussed in the die-off symptoms (page 74). The second, as we mentioned above, is the deficient production of blood by the spleen, providing less blood for the brain.

But there is a third one! With most of the Candida patients, I observed neck pains due to muscle spasms. When you say "muscle spasms," you refer in Acupuncture to excessive energy in the liver-organ. The emotions linked to this organ are anger, irritability and frustration! And, do you know of any Candida patient who has not these emotions in storage? Rejection, being laughed at, subjected at modern torture such as electro shocks, have instilled most patients with these emotions. The spasms on their turn, will again decrease the flow of the posterior circulation to the brain. Acupuncture, acupressure or chiropractic adjustments will be the answer.

Is this disease contagious? Only when there are active lesions in the mouth (trush) or in the vagina. Otherwise, there is no danger of passing this debilitating disease over to your family or friends.

But, it is socially contagious! Let me explain this. Once one of the partners suffers from Candida, the other partner becomes almost immediately a victim. There are so many restrictions, diet wise, most patients become sensitive to perfumes, ink, smoke, gasoline fumes, ... that it is almost impossible for that couple to socialize. This often leads to tension, anger, frustration and rejection, all emotions that are fuel for the disease. Often, the Candida patient, therefore, has guilt feelings for being "such a pest," hindering the recuperation. This disease is surely a test for the stability of any relationship. So how do we diagnose this giant killer?

4

Diagnosis

The clinical picture is the most important. Having been exposed to triggering factors as explained before, will make the patient think twice about these symptoms. Sad to say, but often the patient thinks about this diagnosis before his doctor does. Still now, 80% of the medical professional community does not even believe in the existence of Systemic Candidiasis, in spite of extensive studies performed in Europe. Often, the patient hears from his doctor: "If you have Systemic Candidiasis, you would be in a hospital!" This might be true for Candida 25 years ago, but we now have a new picture of the same disease. And we helped create it. Filling in a questionnaire and score sheet, mentioning symptoms and triggering factors, will provide the patient with a good indicator about possible yeast infection (see appendix, page 137).

The next step we take: specific blood tests like the Candida Antibody test and the Antigen test.

The whole principle of these tests is that Candida, in normal circumstances, is only present in the gastrointestinal tract. The moment Candida cells arrive in the blood stream, they are recognized as strange objects, hence antibodies are formed. In the Candida Antibody test, three kinds of antibodies are measured: IgM, IgA and IgG. Especially the number of the IgM has to be followed, since it will give us information about the degree of activity of the disease. The number of antibodies measured has to be below 100 for the three kinds of antibodies. There are two drawbacks to this test: antibodies cannot be formed by the patient whose immune system is greatly suppressed (cancer and other far advanced diseases); hence, normal levels can be found when the clinical picture is clearly positive. The second drawback is the waiting period of 14 days before the result is known.

The Latex Agglutination Antigen test, on the other hand, does not rely on the formation of antibodies. Merely, the presence of the Candida in the blood (where it is normally not present), will give us the antigen titers. The result is known after 4 days, and both tests cost approximately the same.

This Latex Agglutination test allows detection of a circulating antigen in patients with Candida Albicans, Candida Tropicalis and Candida Parapsilosis. The inability of the clinician to detect early dissemination (spreading) in the fact of colonization of multiple body sites, often leads to delays in effective treatment with disastrous results. Blood cultures are frequently negative or become positive too late to be of diagnostic use. The lag time required for antibody production in the normal host and the impaired immune system in the immune-suppressed patient, have rendered antibody tests relatively ineffective. Therefore, attention seems to be focused more on these antigen tests. In documented disseminated Candida infection, patients had an antigen titer of 1:4 to 1:32. Antigen levels in healthy individuals and in colonized patients with no clinical signs of infection were not greater than 1:2. This same test can be used as a prognostic tool. In each instance of recovery of these patients after adequate treatment, the antigen titer fell to insignificant levels (lower than 1:2) at the end of the therapy.

Severe setback for both tests is that they do not give us any information about what is going on in the gastrointestinal system. In case of negativity for both the above tests, all we can conclude is that the yeast cells have not spread to the blood stream, but it does not exclude the existence of the disease.

Another test useful in following the progress made by the patient is the Urine Indican Test or the OBERMAYER test. Every Candida patient has a certain degree of mal-absorption and mal-digestion. It is a simple and inexpensive urine test: the essential amino acid, tryptophan, is converted to indole by intestinal cleavage of the tryptophan side chain. The higher production of indicans reflects the bacterial activity in the small and large intestines. After mixing some urine with obermeyer reagent, the color of this mixture is read within ten minutes:

urine color	o (normal)
light blue	1
blue	2
violet	3
jet black	4

It is interesting to see how this test can evolve from plus 4 to zero after a couple of months treatment, allowing the patient and the doctor to test the efficacy of the treatment.

The most recent and promising test for Candida is the Candi-Shere Enzyme ImmunoAssay Test (CEIA). What is this test based on? The Candida cell produces several molecules, playing a role in the production of symptoms. Some of these molecules are alcohols, acetaldehyde and hormonal molecules (estrogen, progesterone, testosterone). These small molecules are directly responsible for the clinical effects of Systemic Candidiasis. Large molecules produced by Candida exert their effects directly and they provide a mechanism for diagnosing the syndrome. One of these molecules is the presence of cytoplasmic proteins. They are the metabolic enzymes of Candida and are normally NOT found OUTSIDE of the candida cell. Hence, they are very valuable to us as diagnostic probes. Due to their hidden position inside the yeast cell, very few people have antibodies against these cytoplasmic proteins unless the people are very heavily colonized or infected with Candida Albicans. Normal, low level colonization of the GI tract does not stimulate detectable levels of circulating antibodies against these antigens. This is a big step forward in the diagnosis of Candida, since detection of any form of Candidiasis has historically been very difficult since even "normal" individuals gave positive tests for antibody.

5

Spreading Mechanism

How does the yeast become systemic, almost invading any other organ?

Normally these yeast cells live in harmony in our gastro-intestinal system (especially in the esophagus, small intestines and feces). They live together with bacteria in a concentration of millions of bacteria versus one Candida. These bacteria form the normal flora of the gastrointestinal tract and inhibit the overgrowth of the Candida. This process is called symbiosis: it is the mutual cohabitation of living organisms with benefit to both. What is this normal intestinal flora? It consists of three parts: the main flora, the accompanying and the residual one. The main flora, Anaerobe bacteria (Bacterium Bifidus and Bacteroides); the secondary one consists of the E. Coli, Enterococci and Lactobacilli; the residual one is composed by yeast cells, Clostridia and Staphylococci. This will become important when we have to replace this destroyed flora: the product that contains most of these bacteria will be the best. Right there the patient will have a guideline as to which "Acidoph-ilus" brand to choose. We have to keep in mind that in case of "Dysbiosis" or disturbed relationship between the body and its physiological flora, especially the Bacterium Bifidum, will be suppressed. Through several causes, discussed previously (Causes and Triggering Factors), the concentration of millions of bacteria versus 1 Candida, changes to 1 bacteria versus millions of Candida cells. In normal circumstances, Candida cells do not leave the gastrointestinal tract and spread in the blood. However, the barrier is broken when there is a concentration of millions of yeast cells. This process is called PERSORPTION. Another spreading mechanism is the invasive growth of mycelia (the "legs" of the Candida cells) in the bowel walls so that the blood and lymph vessels can be reached.

Indeed, the Candida can take two forms: the yeast form, which cannot penetrate the small intestine wall, and the fungus form with its mycelia, invading the wall and spreading to the blood.

From practical experience, we see that the disease becomes almost always systemic after 6 to 12 months. Unfortunately, because of late recognition, this is almost always the case. And, it is this spreading to the blood that we are measuring in our blood tests, while those same lab tests will not give us any indication about the prevalence of the Candida in the gastrointestinal tract.

The organ first invaded is the liver, since the portal vein, the big vessel going to the liver, seems to be the carrier or freeway for our yeast cells. You can already see the detrimental effect this has on the detoxification capacity of the patient, since the liver is THE organ to assist us in this process. From there, the yeast cells easily spread to the lungs, heart and other organs. Volkheimer, a German doctor, used starch particles for his test. These particles were pushed through the intestinal wall and found in the lumen of the lung vessel, proving the process of persorption (test done in 1963).

There is, however, a third way of spreading, as the second story about the babies in the County hospital shows: direct infection. Infection is a real danger in intensive care and in any form of catheterizations: intravenous feeding, bladder catheters, dialysis instruments can be the primary source of Candida.

Another way of direct infection happens during surgery.

In medical literature, we find examples of mycotic (yeast) endocarditis after valve surgery.

6
Therapy

The first and best treatment of any disease is the prevention of it. We have to pay close attention to all the triggering factors. Of course, one that can be found in almost any patient is the over use of antibiotics. We know that antibiotics are almost always prescribed for any infection, viral or bacterial. Doctors and patients have become so adjusted to the use of them, that it is almost prescribed or asked for as a reflex. Often it takes all my eloquence to convince a patient that not only should he not take an antibiotic for viral infections, but that it is hazardous to his health! In almost all the medical histories of my patients, I notice the over use of antibiotics. One of my very first questions is, "When did you feel good for the last time and what happened?": antibiotic intake is very frequently the triggering factor. As we know, it is not the only factor. A doctor who accompanied his wife to my office questioned me about this. He said: "Antibiotics have been in use for 40 years and only now do we see this syndrome." Well, first of all, we probably never recognized the problem before (or even now), but what have we done to our environment, with continuous spraying of chemicals, car exhaust fumes, atomic plants; what have we done to our foods, with preservatives, low dosage antibiotics and hormones ... to say nothing of stress levels in this decade of zombied yuppies, totally sold to the evils of the corporate environment. Do we realize that more than 2000 preservatives are allowed in this country, while only 8 in France, 5 in Belgium and in Sweden, zero is found in the food. I read how a medical doctor in one of his articles is convinced that we still have the best food of the whole world, right here in the USA. I wished it were true. We sure have the basis and ingredients for the healthiest diet, but we sure find ways to mess it up.

Of course, there are enough indications for antibiotic intake. How do we protect ourselves then? By taking from the start, a high dosis of Acidophilus (6 TBS of liquid or four times, a quarter of a teaspoon powder). It is such a pity that most doctors wait for the appearance of diarrhea before suggesting the intake of Acidophilus. And, at that point, mostly in the form of yoghurt, which has a negligible concentration considering the purpose involved. Patients who are at that time on any anti-fungal medication should increase their dosage for the length of the antibiotic intake. Even for those patients who have not taken any medication, a low dosage of an anti-fungal medication intake is advised. (See: Kill Candida)

Cortisone, the "pill," and immunosuppressive medications should be avoided if at all possible. Hypothyroidism, diabetes mellitus and anemia are checked and, if positive, corrected.

Yeast containing foods have to be avoided totally in the beginning of the therapy. I remember a patient in my practice who used to perspire heavily and had a very low degree of energy. In fact, as he would leave my treatment table, his body would stick to the paper, he was perspiring so much. A mere seven-day anti-yeast diet completely changed this picture. More about the diet will be discussed further.

It is also obvious that most patients of this type have to change their life styles. We have to realize that the changes have to come from within ourselves; a doctor is only there to give some guidelines. It is a bad start if we reason like one of my patients: "I give YOU one year to change me." I personally will not change anybody. Nobody

can rescue you if there is not the determination and perse-
verance to want a healthier life. Because that is what your
reward is. And, do not believe those who say: "If I have to
live this way, I would rather live a shorter life." Our
survival instinct is our strongest instinct. What those
people actually hope is that they can get away with abusing
their bodies. Do not fall into this trap of denial! Five
thousand years ago the Chinese already knew that worry and
obsession about the past will injure the spleen and decrease
its energy. People with Candidiasis unfortunately, or should
I say logically, most always fall into this category. They
are mostly intelligent, very analytical and have an obsessive
compulsive nature. Because of the rejection that they all
encounter, worry and frustration are constant growing
feelings, starting the vicious cycle of spleen depression:
the more they worry, the less energy is in the spleen, and
the less energy, the more they will worry! And, that's where
support groups can do a marvelous job. Finding people who
have gone through the same suffering will convince Candida
patients that: one, they are not crazy and, two, there is
hope for recovery. Almost all patients are in a different
stage of the disease and could give advise on how they
oversee their darkest moments. In the same way that the AA
movement is more successful in supporting alcoholics and cure
alcoholism than any hospital treatment, support groups will,
in the future, be a cornerstone in overcoming this terrible
disease. While going through a change of life style, it is a
good opportunity to initiate psycho-therapy and resolve all
the issues left over from childhood. A good counselor will
help deal with frustration, depression, mood swings, suicidal
thoughts and above all, give you the attention you deserve,
without judgment. Denial, misplacement and anger are frequently found in Candida patients. I remember a patient who
was overweight and full of yeast; she could not bring herself
to eat more healthily. She bought all the wrong foods for
the rest of the family and "because she could not let the

food spoil," she participated (probably gladly) in this diet. Who was she fooling here? A list of support groups and competent counselors is added at the end of the book.

As we have mentioned before, another triggering factor is the **humidity and presence of molds.** They will decrease the energy in the spleen. How to protect ourselves? Start eliminating dampness in your home by checking the walls and roof for leaks. Waterproof walls and ceilings before painting. Paint, instead of wallpapering, to avoid the growth of molds. Avoid carpets as floor covering but replace them with wood floors, vinyl or ceramic tile. Molds grow in carpet while the dust is trapped in the carpet, causing allergic reactions. Allow good air circulation in closets by leaving space between hanging clothes. Check especially leather clothing, belts, shoes and luggage since molds have a tendency to grow on these items. Keep bathrooms and laundry rooms well aired: spread out towels and washcloths for fast drying. In fact, in humid conditions, use air conditioning or a dehumidifier: molds hate dry environments. And, of course, avoid foods which contain molds or are related to molds (mushrooms).

Sometimes, the problem caused by presence of molds can be so bad, that there is nothing left to do but move. I know of a family that moved to three different states before they settled down in an "ecological" house, free of carpets, gas stove and surrounded by woods, away from traffic. In the process, the husband lost his job and the whole family was isolated. Not everybody wants to make this sacrifice. It is easier when you live in a rental house, but what do you do when you live in an expensive house along a foggy beach and your partner is healthy. There will be a lot of anger, frustration and despair for such patients because they are trapped in a predicament: it is too expensive to move, the partner does not want to move, and each time the patient enters the house, the symptoms are aggravated after one hour. These are not isolated cases, and they are hard to resolve!

The problem of being sensitive to the environment, for many patients, goes beyond the mold sensitivity. A great many women have become chemically sensitive to the fumes from gas stoves. In fact, gas is a major culprit, and I would advise anyone, especially Candida patients, to remove all the gas lines and replace the stove with an electric one.

It is a good idea to avoid airborne chemicals in the home, such as waxes, mothballs, glue or anything else that evaporates.

Avoid paint and varnish removers because of the presence of benzene, linked to leucemia, after long-time exposure. Severe setbacks in Candida patients can be seen after exposure to freshly painted rooms. It is best to avoid sleeping in them and move if you can to a friend's house for at least a couple of days. In fact, it is best to paint in the spring, so that we can leave the windows open for the rest of the summer. Candida patients will detect paint fumes for three months after application.

Where are some of the favorite places for molds? Basement, kitchen and bathroom are harboring molds in great quantities. Be sure to throw out those piles of old newspapers, magazines, clothes and leftovers, carpets and pillows. A favorite place in the bathroom is between the tiles and caulking. The overall solution is a built-in shower exhaust. Be sure to check the surplus water tray on self-defrosting refrigerators. The growth of these molds on their favorite places is enhanced during the warm, humid summer months: spores are sent throughout the house when the molds mature.

A natural anti-mold to sprinkle in places of mold growth is Borax, an efficient mold growth retardant. Another efficient anti-mold product is formaldehyde (37% solution), available in any pharmacy under the name "Formaline." Put one inch of Formaline in a container. Candida patients should leave their homes for 48 hours while the Formaline is working. Upon their return, they should air the house out.

One container per 12 x 12 foot space will do the job!

Unfortunately, I have in my practice some patients who are not just having the problem with Candida, EBV, CMV, ... they seem to be allergic to 20th century life. All they can do is pack up their belongings and move into the desert to avoid pollution, synthetics and the likes. But I believe there is another way out; namely, following a strict way of life for a certain time (mostly one month). It is outlined below.

Upon rising at your SET time, drink at least 2 glasses of water with the juice of one lemon (the ideal detoxifier!) Take at this moment, 8-12 tablets of wheat grass, 1-2 teaspoons liquid garlic (Kyolic) and 1/2 tsp. megadophilus.

Spend at least one hour in a brisk walk, biking, jogging or any other outdoor activity. Practice breathing deeply. Be sure to start out slowly, each day increasing your pace. Shower with warm water, finish with cold.

At your SET breakfast time, mix 2 tbs. of psyllium seeds with 4 oz. of water or pineapple juice or papaya juice. Wash a bundle of parsley, mix it in your blender with just enough unsweetened pineapple juice to break it down to a nice thick drink. In case of stomach irritation of hyperacidity, use fresh cabbage juice (8 oz.) right out of the juicer and before each meal.

For seven days your diet should be only beans (pinto, kidney, lentils, navy) and greens (any, such as leaf lettuce, celery, avocado, peas, spinach, diced young turnips cooked with turnip greens, kale, collard). Cooking greens with chopped onions and garlic makes a tasty side dish. Steam all your salads and vegetables; they are better tolerated this way.

Beans are to be washed, placed in a kettle with water to cover and bring to boil for 10 minutes. Drain, place back in the kettle with fresh water and bring to a boil again, repeating this process three times. Place long cooking beans (navy, pinto, ...) in a slow cooker after boiling and cook on high for 12 HOURS, using one large onion, one bulb of garlic, a little sea salt and cayenne.

Vary the beans toward the fifth day by adding garden tomatoes, watch for any reaction. Rice crackers with avocado for spread may be used the first week.

Take you Kyolic and megadophilus after each meal. If you wish to have three meals, your meal times should be 6 a.m., 1 p.m. and 5:30 p.m. The ideal is two meals with nothing after 3 p.m. The third meal must follow the principals, only fruit and grains are allowed in the evening. Mainly pineapple, avocado, apricots, papaya, if they do not contain artificial sweeteners.

The MOST important facet in this "cave man" diet is plenty of water! In the early morning, fill a quart jar and by the time you retire at night, you should have drunk 3 quarts of water. Do not drink water with your meals, neither 20 minutes before or 1 hour after meals.

Candida sufferers all need some help with digestion: Bromelain (GRL), 2 tablets with each meal is an excellent help. Other supplements for these patients are L-Tryptophan, a valuable sleep aid, taken 1 hour before going to bed adding a complex carbohydrate (banana). Together with another amino acid, Thyrosin 500 mg., it is the ideal way to fight depression and mood swings.

Goats milk is very valuable for high quality absorption. It has been found especially valuable with those suffering from allergies. It has a calming effect on the most nervous individual. Some 4 oz. before you exercise helps down the garlic, 4 oz. at meals with 8 oz. before retiring benefits those losing weight.

Fruits, vegetables, nuts and grains make the ideal diet. From too much sugar in our usual "junk" diet, our body has a hard time in the beginning handling the natural sugars in high sugar fruits. For this reason, pineapple, grapefruit, lemon and avocado seem to be the only ones tolerated the first week. The other fruits should be added very slowly and best peel your fruit (except if it is organic). Start adding grain the second week to avoid allergic reactions. Do not eat sweet vegetables such as corn and potatoes together, at least not in the beginning. All meat and animal products are hard to digest, contain no fiber and are unnecessary at this moment in your diet.

It is extremely important to use up to 8 tsp. of Kyolic; gradually, you will be able to cut down to 6 and 4 tsp. A good combination is 6 tsp. Kyolic with 6 tablets of Kyolic.

As you can see, this diet is no easy way, but life for those poor patients is never easy. They are allergic to practically every food, supplement, cigarette smoke, household cleansers, plants (because of the soil the plants are in, great place for molds!). Going into stores is impossible, they can only wear 100% cotton clothes, and perfumes literally kill them. Gas fumes from other cars induce asthma attacks and swollen throats.

It is frightening that the food we eat, the water we drink, medicine we take, clothing we wear, as well as the air we breath at home, work or school, constitute not only our environment, but in many cases, becoming a real menace to our physical and mental well being. What can we do to stay healthy in a chemical world?

Good health is not a gift, it is something we must help search for and find. As chronic illness overtakes us, basic rules become more and more important: eat organically, read the labels, eat less sugar and salt, and bring a variety of fruit and vegetables to our diet.

Sixty percent of the leading causes of death are linked to our over-consumption of fats, cholesterol, sugar, salt and alcohol. Cutting off the fat on our meat will already avoid most of the chemicals. As mentioned before, chickens are fed antibiotics, cattle and hogs are given hormones. These powerful chemicals end up in our bodies in such high levels that they can be measured in laboratories. Be aware of fish as a meat substitute since preservatives are often added at sea to keep fish fresh until it can be brought to the processor. Fish caught in colder climates where this is not needed are safer. Prefer the Icelandic and Canadian ones. A frightening example is the following. One of my Candida patients bought some orange roughy. As I advised her to keep a diary of everything she was eating, she discovered that she reacted violently after the consumption of this fish. When she asked the vendor, he replied that "many people seem to have that reaction" and that it comes from a preservative "Hoplasthethus Atlanticus," added to the fish the moment it is caught. It is a fish caught in Australia and New Zealand, therefore, needs this preservative. Trout is another fish frequently treated with preservatives. The best fish to buy is salmon, halibut and rock cod, all caught in cold waters.

Remember also that "natural" is NOT organic. Only food grown without commercial sprays and fertilizers can be labeled organic. Unless food is labeled organic, you should not be paying more for it. Statements such as "No chemicals or preservatives added" on labels mean often that food was commercially grown.

Call your Department of Health and ask what additives are in the local water supply. These additives are often a source of sensitivity. Use water bottled in glass, not plastic. If the best you can drink is bottled in plastic, pour it into a glass sterile jar and leave the lid off a while so plastic can gas out.

Some other handy advise in your kitchen:
. Use stainless steel, iron, glass or porcelain-like cookware since non-stick pans are bad contaminators (petro-lined!).
. Cook organic beans in a slow cooker.
. Rotate foods by spacing each one five days apart. By spacing these foods, you are actually performing the most simple allergy test. You eliminate a certain food (wheat, milk, corn, beef, ...) for four days, eat it on the fifth day and observe any adverse reactions. Under these specific conditions, adverse reactions are noted within minutes.

. Cooking sometimes makes food more tolerable for the highly sensitive. You can freeze leftovers and eat them five days later.

. Try fasting for 24 hours. If this is difficult, it is almost certain that you have some important food allergies.

As the illness grows, you become addicted to smoking, alcohol and drugs. Food you become allergic to can do the same things. They too can fool you into thinking you need them. Sugar is the best example. After consuming it, for an hour or two you might feel better (relieving the apparent hypoglycemia), even though it is the source of your problem. When you will remove an important food that acts as an adverse reactor, you will experience withdrawal symptoms. But feel good about it, you discovered this "masking" enemy because removing it from your diet will make a big difference in how you feel. And, in case you are a "universal" reactor or allergic to all foods, clinical ecologists now have neutralization techniques which make it possible for the extremely ill people to eat almost normally. One of the techniques is the fenolic food testing.

It is wise to avoid those who smoke or wear hairspray or perfumes. Wash your clothes without detergents but use mild soap, borax and soda in the laundry. Wash windows with vinegar water. And, above all, develop a sense of humor and guard against self-pity! Learn to listen to your body because environmental illness will affect each individual in its own way.

There is another important factor for these "super-allergic" people: positive ions. Ions are submicroscopic particles that have no taste and don't stimulate our other sense organs in any other way. Positive ions are produced by heating air, by air moving past an obstruction such as a bend in an air conditioning duct, by snythetic fabrics and are easily found in crowds of people. Do you recognize this situation? This is exactly what we find in most of the modern buildings, from our workplaces to our homes.

Negative ions on the other hand, seem to be the most beneficial ions (it is the extra electron that makes them negative). Where do we find these ions? Falling water is a natural source of negative ions and we all remember the good feelings associated with showers, or being in the neighborhood of the ocean or waterfalls. Unfortunately, the positive ions have a strong hold in nature too; they are associated with the "named" winds around the world: "Santa Ana" in Southern California, the "Foehn" in Europe and the "Sharav" in Israel. At least 30% of the world population is suffering from these weather related conditions.

As research continued, it was found that humans produce a hormone called SEROTONINE under the stress of too many positive ions. What does serotonine do? It is a neurotransmitter, involved in the induction of sleep, in other words, we need some amount of it to induce our sleep. However, we can already see the disastrous consequences when too much of this serotonin is formed: we will seem sleepy and without energy all the time. Extreme fatigue, depression, irritability and decreased breathing capacity are present in all of these patients. And, I am sure you have heard the word "lunatic". They are those hyperactive people swinging to deep depressions. This situation becomes a little more understandable when we know that the general charge on earth is negative, while the charge in the atmosphere is positive. This positive ion layer sends its ions down to our level when it is moved tidally by the gravitational effect of the moon: the result is an increase in positive ions, with disastrous consequences for the weather sensitive people.

So should we only breath negative ions? In general, they have no side-effects, but depressed levels of serotonin as would be the case, would lead to insomnia and hyper-alertness. This hyper-yang stage will not allow any cell repair and disturb the natural organ clock. But being exposed to an air ionizer, even the whole day, will not have that negative effect. Quite to the contrary, you will have added protection against viruses and bacteria since they will be pulled out of the air, simply like other dust particles.

Once we have taken care of the triggering factors, we will start our battle against Candidiasis. And, it is a severe battle requiring all the troops that we have available. Seven major steps will win this fight: 1) **STARVE THE CANDIDA**; 2) **KILL THE CANDIDA**; 3) **EVACUATE THE DEAD CANDIDA OR TOXINS**; 4) **AVOID SPREADING TO THE BLOOD STREAM (SYSTEMIC CANDIDIASIS)**; 5) **REPLACE THE NORMAL FLORA**; 6) **BOOST THE IMMUNE SYSTEM**; 7) **REPLACE THE MISSING SUPPLEMENTS**. Step by step, we will discuss each of these weapons against yeast. It has amazed me time and time again, that people do, for instance, three steps well, but pay no attention to the other ones. Inevitably, they will miss on the curing of the disease, arrive at a plateau in their healing or delay the recovery of this debilitating disease.

A. The Anti Yeast Diet

The first line of defense against Candida is diet. Diet has always been and should be the starting point of a healthy life. In ancient China they had different classes of doctors. The highest in esteem was the nutritional doctor since he prevented the disease from appearing. The one lowest in esteem was the doctor who took care of the patient once the disease had already appeared. This is exactly what the majority of the present doctors do. And, it does not look like any improvement is in sight: insurance companies do not pay for inexpensive preventive medicine, but see no problem with reimbursing the multi-million dollar bills from hospitals. I read in a medical magazine an interview with a Nobel price winner in Medicine: she claimed that the importance of food is highly exaggerated and plays a minimal role in maintaining our health. I am sorry to say so, but my grandmother had more common sense. Food is still the fuel that your motor will run on, and if I have the choice, I prefer to go for quality!

Diet is very important, and at the same time, very difficult and frustrating. However, if a patient feels that s/he does not make any progress or comes to a plateau during the treatment, the first reflex has to be a closer look at the food intake. Many times, a patient thinks s/he is eating all the right things, but upon closer examination, many foods cause yeast growth. Therefore, the patient does not make any breakthrough and returns to his previous bad eating habits, since "this boring diet does not make any difference." And, s/he promptly rewards himself with ice cream and cake: the rest is history, and Candida wins the game!

Each time I start explaining the content of this diet, I will invariably hear: "I may as well starve, there is nothing more left to eat." Maybe so at first sight. What it really requires for most people is a total change from their convenient junk food diet to one that requires more imagination and work. And forget parties and eating out. That's why this disease is such an isolating disease; the patient actually transmits the disease over to the partner. The partner becomes a prisoner of the house, since the Candida patient can't go out, cannot go to movies or parties because of environmental factors. Of course, this is not always taken in gratitude! And the poor Candida patient receives more rejection, anger and impatience. And the vicious cycle is closed: many of these patients have an enormous amount of anger and frustration, something they can best deal with in a support group, led by a competent psychologist.

Basically, the diet is LOW in carbohydrates (CBH) and HIGH in proteins. Before going into detail, some important facts have to be pointed out.

First, avoid raw and cold foods! Climactic dampness spells doom for the spleen; the cold and raw food causes INTERIOR dampness. The moment we see "damp," we know it means trouble for the spleen. I have seen patients in my office who could not lose weight despite being on what they thought was a healthy diet. They were only eating salads (our daily salad bar!) and raw vegetables and could not lose one pound and even gained weight. So limit salads and totally avoid raw vegetables for the time being.

Secondly, do not eat leftovers. Being in the refrigerator, the molds have a great opportunity to grow over night! Freeze your leftovers and reheat them.

Thirdly, ROTATE your foods. The easiest way to acquire allergies to food is to eat the same things over and over. Examples of rotation diets are outlined further in the book.

Furthermore, if you start this diet, do it a hundred percent! Doing it halfway will only give you headaches, frustration and anger. You will not make any progress, your yeast cells will keep on growing; so will your cravings and all the other symptoms for that matter.

As we have already mentioned, the increased growth of yeast before the menstrual cycle due to progesterone, yeast intake has to be extremely well watched around this period. Try to exercise, treat yourself to something pleasant (nature walks, a movie if you can, or a phone call to a good friend who can give you some support).

And, last but not least, this is not a diet for the rest of your life. Do not think you will never be able to touch cheese, dairy products or breads again. The better start you give yourself, the shorter this period will be. Usually, I say to the patient: "Try it very strictly for seven days." Everybody can do it for that period and usually it will be enough for a major change in the patient's symptoms. Once s/he feels the benefit of his diet change, s/he is positively stimulated to go on with it. As the patient gets better, blood "allergies" will disappear, s/he will be able to add new foods week by week, and gradually break away from a monotonous diet.

The quickest way to recovery is to follow this diet as well as possible for one month. After this period, certain foods will be re-introduced one by one: this way, we will recognize an "allergic" reaction right away. If your body at that moment is not balanced out, you will react on that particular food within a half an hour. Mostly, you will experience headaches, bloating and sudden fatigue. The same happens when patients are "cheating" on their diet. Some of the foods that can be tried first will be some cereals, maybe some rye, some more fruits, oatmeals. But please stay away for a longer time from wines, champagne, dairy products and, of course, SUGAR. You want to visualize what happens in your gastrointestinal system when you add sugar? When you bake bread and you add the cube of yeast to dissolve in the 115 degree water, nothing happens. The moment you add sugar to this mixture, it starts growing, bubbling, the smell is more activated and it warms up. Can you image this all happening in your poor bowels? No wonder, bloating and gas are an immediate reaction. On the other hand, cheating once on your diet does NOT put you automatically back where you started from. Merely, you will go through some die-off, sign of the continuous battle between the yeast and your defenders.

And do not forget that at some point in your diet, you will crave the very foods that created the condition. If you understand that you desire the very thing that is being eliminated, you can better overcome that pressing craving. One has to be clear in his commitment to healing and take an honest look at the payoff he is getting from being sick.

1. Forbidden foods or yeast foods

Breads which are almost always craved by Candida patients are a big no-no. And this includes Wheat, as well as Rye breads (even if yeast-free)! Other main culprits are: dairy products, cheese of all kinds, cottage cheese, mushrooms (this is a fungus!), wine and champagne. Other yeast containing foods are:

apple - pear - grapes - vinegar - condiments (except pepper, paprika, onion and garlic) - salad dressing (except oil and lemon) - tomato sauce - barbecue sauce - teas (including ALL herbal teas!) - coffee (including decaf) - whiskey - cognac- oatmeals - cereals - horseradish - cookies - cakes - honey- sugar - Nutrasweet - fruit juices - ice cream - almost any fruit (except some tropical ones) - dry fruits.

Some of the above nutrients do not contain yeasts but they will enhance the growth of the yeast cells.

High carbohydrate foods are also to be limited: lima beans, white potatoes, winter squash, lentils, popcorn, pumpkin, peas and barley.

2. Allowed foods

This is the return to our plain water. Sometimes it is very advantageous to add lemon juice (five drops in a glass of water) in order to free the body from the dead toxins.

Only two teas are allowed: the first one is Taheebo tea or Pau D'Arco tea, a Brazilian herbal tea. This tea is known to have natural anti-fungal properties. Two to three cups daily (not more in order to avoid too heavy a die-off) will often clear the head. To improve its taste, lemon or cinnamon can be added. Another important tea is the black walnut tea, known for its eliminating effects of worms and parasites, frequently seen in Candida patients.

In case of constipation, papaya juice can be allowed. It is beneficial to mix a glass half of water with a glass half of papaya juice.

Special attention must be paid to CRANBERRY juice, sometimes referred to as 'nature's healing cocktail'. Cystitis-like symptoms are a frequent symptom with Candida patients. For more than fifty years, cranberry products have been used in our diets to control the growth of bacteria in the urine and also to reduce strong odor in urine. Cranberry is a native American product that is used traditionally to make sauces and drinks. This fruit is very acidic so that its juice is not easily taken as nature provides it. To improve the taste, the juice is customarily diluted with water. Cranberry juice concentrate is available in health food stores. This product is natural cranberries diluted with water and does not contain added sugar or sweeteners. Another form, available in health food stores, is the cranberry juice concentrate in soft gelatin capsules. Cranberries are a source of Vitamins A, C, B-complex and several minerals such as potassium, manganese, iron and calcium. It is a strong inhibitor of bacterial adherence which prevents foreign invading bacteria from attaching to the urinary tract lining.

3. Other allowed foods

Corn - Popcorn - Rice (by preference, brown rice and wild rice) - eggs, rice cakes - buckwheat - millet - amaranth (cereal and seeds) - gooseberries - all fresh meats (except BEEF and PORK) - all seafood - all vegetables (steamed or stir-fried) - all nuts, unsalted, raw (except peanuts and pistachios) - all seeds - salads with oil and lemon (as salad dressing) - yams - beans - butter - nut butters (except peanut) - rice bran - brown rice cream - condiments (see rotation diet) - quinoa (keenwa) - rice noodle - Japanese buckwheat noodles - goats milk - tropical fruits (pineapple, papaya, mango, kiewi, banana, berries, honeydew melon, but no cantelope or watermelon, guava, lemons) - wheatgrass juice- corn tortillas - corn chips - goat cheese.

4. Key foods profile

POPCORN

What's fun to make, low in calories, does not cause cavities, is economical and good for you? Popcorn, truly an all-American discovery. It is a type of corn with small hard kernels. The plants have the same food values as other varieties of corn. Each kernel contains about 13% moisture which will change to steam when heated to 400.F. A cup of buttered popcorn has about 40 calories. It is part of a balanced diet and not a junk food at all. Even a little drizzled with butter, it has only 65 calories compared to 200 calories for four chocolate chip cookies. According to the American Dental Association, popcorn does not contribute to cavities: it is a safe and nutritious snack. In fact, it may help teeth and gums because of its cleansing and massaging effect. It is also high in fiber, adding bulk to the diet thus preventing constipation, some chronic diseases of the large intestines and decreasing the appetite by causing a filled-up feeling. Fiber in the diet is also believed to protect against colon cancer.

BEANS

Everyone seems interested in them these days. They are an excellent source of protein and have a longer shelf-life than most animal, vegetable and fruit products. They contain no cholesterol and 80% less total fat than lean beef. They are an excellent source of minerals. Cooking beans is a little complex. They require long cooking times. One way to decrease the cooking time is to presoak the beans, either overnight or plunge them into boiling water for two minutes and then soak them for one hour. After this, beans need to be simmered for 2 hours to make them tender enough to eat. Beans are an excellent low-fat source of protein and combined with rice or corn, they serve as the primary protein source for much of the world's population. One of the problems with eating beans is that they cause gas in most individuals. This depends on the non-digestible carbohydrates in the beans which are fermented by bacteria and yeasts. If you like beans, but have problems with gas (which most Candida patients have), activated charcoal can help. Twenty to fifty grams taken orally can decrease the amount of gas in the large intestine.

What are other gas producing foods? apples, bananas, brussel sprouts, broccoli, cauliflower, celery, milk products, onions, raisins, prunes and wheat germ.

RICE

Rice is truly one of the world's great treasures. For more than half the earth's population, rice is the staff of life. Asia produces more than 90% of the world's rice. In warm, wet climates, rice can be grown continuously and yields from 100 to 200 pounds per acre. Newly harvested rice is covered by an unedible husk which is removed from the dried grains by pounding and shaking. What remains is brown rice. If the kernels are then rubbed until the bran is removed, we have white polished rice. The bran coating on brown rice contains many ingredients, which can be critical where rice is a major source of calories.

It is the LEAST allergenic of all grains. Wheat triggers four times as many allergic reactions, corn three times as many. Washing or soaking rice removes the B vitamins.

AMARANTH

Amaranth, a little-known crop of the Americas, is grown either as a grain crop or as a leafy vegetable. Despite its obscurity, it offers important promise for feeding the world's hungry. This broad-leafed plant is one of the few non-grasses that produce significant amounts of edible "cereal" grain. It grows vigorously, resisting drought, heat and pests. It is a beautiful crop with brilliantly colored leaves, stems and flowers. The seed heads occur in massive numbers, sometimes more than 50,000 to a plant. Amaranth has two big advantages: it has a very high protein content, 16 percent, compared to the 12% of wheat, 7-10% of rice and 9% of maize. Later, it was found that the seed contains protein of unusual quality. It is high in the amino acid lysine. Therefore, it is a nutritional complement to conventional cereals. Different recipes of cooking with amaranth are found at the end of the book. When heated, the tiny amaranth grains pop and taste like a nut-flavored popcorn and can be eaten as a snack. When amaranth flour is mixed with corn flour, the combination reaches the perfect 100 score, because the amino acids that are deficient in one are abundant in the other one: amaranth is high in lysine and tryptophan, corn high in leucine.

GOOSEBERRIES

Calcium deficiency, a condition that often manifests itself by osteoporosis of the bones and poor mineralization of the teeth, has an excellent natural remedy. It is gooseberries. 100 grams or 35 ounces of gooseberries contain 564 mgs of calcium, an extraordinary amount considering that in the same amount of apples, there is 8 mgs. of calcium, 52 in dates and 116 to 175 in cow's milk.

At first thought, it would seem that the people in this country, given their relatively high consumption of milk and other dairy products, would easily get all the calcium their systems need from their daily fare. But alas, that is not so.

Only about 10% of elements in the cow's milk purchased at your supermarket can be readily assimilated. Of course, for a Candida patient, the problem becomes even more acute: dairy products are out. Hence, the vogue for calcium pills, which are selling so well at drug and health food stores. The usual dose is one gram of calcium per day, of which at most 100 mg. will be bioavailable. Compare that to the 200 grams of gooseberries: the amount of calcium will be 1.28 grams, all of it bioavailable.

The plant was introduced to Western Europe by Anne of Russia. Gooseberries were her beauty and health secret. A French clinician who has studied and used food plants in his medical practice for many ailments that do not respond to drugs, wrote that gooseberries are a good appetizer, good for the digestion, a natural laxative in sufficient quantities and a diuretic.

QUINOA (pronounced KEENWA)

It is one of the "rediscovered" foods. Quite similar in properties to Amaranth. It is a grain that comes from the Andean Mountain regions of South America. Its origin is ancient: it was one of the three staple foods (along with corn and potatoes) of the Inca civilization. It is respect-fully known as the Mother Grain.

It contains more protein than any other grain: an average of 6%. Quinoa is, in fact, a complete protein, with an essential amino acid balance close to the ideal. It is high in lysine, methionine and cystine, thus boosting the food value of other grains when combined with them. Although no single food can supply all of the life-sustaining nutrients, quinoa comes closer than any other food.

And, if this is not enough, listen to the following advantages. It is light, tasty and easy to digest. Its flour is low in gluten: it can be used in all baking goods. It is easy and quick to prepare: a whole dish takes just 15 minutes to prepare. It is perfect in the summertime: Quinoa's lightness, combined with its versatility in cold dishes like salads and desserts, make it an ideal source of good warm weather nutrition. Cooked quinoa expands almost five times compared to about three times for brown rice. It is an excellent source of nutrition for kids and nursing mothers.

Recipes with Quinoa are written down in the food section, page #155 .

NUTS AND SEEDS

There is a growing evidence that seeds and nuts were the major staples of early humans. Archaeological excavations show that prehistoric men and women frequently used the seeds and nuts of a wide variety of wild plants, especially in the northern climates. The season during which food could be gathered was short, and as seeds and nuts are easily storable, they were no doubt a stable and convenient food source. As agriculture began, an advanced type of seed, the cereal grains, has replaced nuts in importance. Still, highly nutritious nuts are used as "famine foods" by many cultures and, even today, many primitive people depend upon seeds and nuts for a large part of their nourishment. For the Candida patient, it provides an excellent snack, as long as they are eaten UNSALTED and raw, or at least not honey roasted. What are the nuts and seeds available?

Let's start with the no-no's. Two nuts to avoid are peanuts and pistachios. The peanut is not a nut, rather it is a legume or bean. Peanuts are mainly grown for their oil, except in the USA where 50 percent of the crop going into peanut butter. Peanuts are susceptible to the aflatoxin mold, one of the most powerful carcinogens known. Roasting does not destroy the mold, therefore, natural foods manufacturers retest them before using in peanut butter. Because of its moldy content, peanuts are out for the Candida patient.

The pistachios are the seeds of an evergreen which is grown in the Mediterranean for over 5000 years. They are usually dyed white or red for eye appeal, although natural foods stores don't find this treatment appealing and stock only the undyed ones. Since they are salted and roasted exclusively, this excludes them for the yeast diet.

Chestnuts are allowed only in small quantities: they are low in calories, but also low in protein and high in starch or carbohydrates. They should be eaten fresh or boiled but not dried as it makes them sweeter.

Pinenuts, coming from the Mediterranean and China, contain

more protein than any other nut. They are high priced ($7 per pound), and have a definite piney taste. One of the most popular nuts in the natural foods store is the walnut. Their probable origin is Persia, although they have been under cultivation for so many centuries that their exact place of origin is unknown. Some walnuts are darker than others; the dark ones were grown on the side of the tree that received more sunshine. But outside color is not as important as the color inside which should be white and clean. Most natural foods stores buy lower grade nuts, which have no need for perfect cosmetic appearance.

Hazelnuts are another delicious treat. They are often used as a symbol of love. They are the most common nut tree in England and Spain. They have a pleasant taste, and their small round shape makes them easy and fun to eat.

Almonds are the oldest and most widely grown of all nuts. It is very closely related to the peach. Most of the almonds used in the USA are grown in California, therefore, organic almonds are rarely seen outside of California. Their shells protect the nut against oxidation and rancidity. Good almonds have a smooth and even shape with intact skin. Almonds become more digestible after roasting; raw they should be eaten in small quantities.

Cashews are the fruit of a tropical evergreen, originally from Brazil. Traditionally, the fruits were picked by hand and the nuts removed and dried in the sun, then placed among burning logs where the heat would crack them open. The 45% fat content makes them hard to store, while raw tend to be indigestible. Dry-roasted cashews, therefore, became increasingly more popular.

SEEDS are another delicious snack for Candida patients: **sesame seeds, sunflower seeds** and **pumpkin seeds**. Sesame is the oldest known herb grown for its seeds. They are extremely nutritious and higher versatile. Five thousand years ago, the Chinese had already gone beyond merely eating them and burned the oil to make soot for ink blocking.

Nutritionally, sesame seeds are real power houses. They contain over 35% protein and have twice as much calcium as milk. Since dairy products are out for Candida patients, these seeds are a welcome source for much needed calcium. Most of the seeds used in natural foods stores come from Central America.

Sunflower seeds were used extensively by the American Indians - made into bread and blended in drinks. They are nutritionally similar to sesame seeds but are even higher in protein and phosphorus, although they have less calcium. Fluorine, Vitamins D, E and B-complex are other plus points. The important thing about these seeds is to check their cleanliness: they should be firm, not too hard with few broken seeds.

Pumpkin seeds are highly nutritious since they contain up to 30% protein; they played an important role in the diets of North American indians.

MILLET

This is the ideal grain for the Candida patient. As stressed before, the root of the problem is a deficiency of energy in the Spleen-Pancreas. Millet is said to be good for the Spleen and Stomach (the Yin-Yang unit), and because of its alkaline nature, it is good for people who suffer from acidosis. It is considered to have the most complete protein of all the grains and high in minerals. The variety sold in health foods stores here is the pearl millet.

SWEETENERS

One thing that everyone agrees upon is that white sugar be removed from the diet. As soon as we decided to give up this poison, we began searching for "natural" alternatives that can satisfy our sweet tooth. Unfortunately, no such sweetener exists. We should keep in mind that there is no evidence that the use of sweeteners is necessary to maintain health. On the other hand, sugar intake is linked to arthritis, hypertension, obesitas, diabetes and dental caries. Unfortunately, Americans today consume over fifteen times the sugar they did 100 years ago.

All sweeteners are concentrated simple sugars and as such, cannot be considered whole foods. Natural sweeteners have many of the same effects on the body as white sugar. Common sense tells us that if we eat whole foods, the vitamins, minerals and enzymes present will allow smooth metabolism of the sugars contained therein. The best way for the body to take in sugar is through the digestion of complex carbohydrates: the starch from grains, vegetables and fruits is digested slowly, releasing sugar into the blood gradually. This prevents the insulin overload and adrenal exhaustion that accompanies the ingestion of concentrated simple sugars. It is evident that the Candida patient get his sweet taste from tropical fruits such as pineapple, papaya, mango, banana, honeydew melon and kiewi. They are best eaten once a day, not combined with any other food: they make the ideal breakfast. Do not eat fruit the whole day, since the amount of sugar will be too much. Do not eat dried fruits since the main sugar in dried pineapple, for instance, is sucrose: it may even amount to over 50% of the product. Another important aspect of the tropical fruits is their content in digestive enzymes: papain and bromelain are two powerful enzymes, found in papaya and pineapple. Especially the first month of the diet, molasses, honey, corn syrup, maple syrup, malt syrup and even amasake are no-no's for the Candida patient. Amasake is nothing else but cooked rice or barley inoculated with the Aspergillus MOLD! From all these sweetners, maple syrup is the most organic and can be introduced into the diet after one month.

5. Example of food rotation

DAY ONE	DAY TWO	DAY THREE	DAY FOUR
Watercress	Brussel Sprouts	Cabbage	Chives
Artichoke	Endive	Iceberg lettuce	Green pepper
Parsley	Romaine Lettuce	Spinach	Beets
Asparagus	Broccoli	Celery	Sweet potato
Leeks	Corn	Alfalfa sprouts	White potato
Avocado	Zucchini	Cucumber	Egg white
Yellow squash	Eggplant	Pumpkin	Calves liver
Carrots	Onions	Turnips	Anchovy
Tomatoes	Chicken	Duck	Lobster
Radish	Turkey	Lamb	Salmon
Beef	Cod	Veal	Shrimp
Egg Yolk	Halibut	Crab	Tuna
Pork	Scallops	Herring	Lima beans
Clam	Swordfish	Red Snapper	String beans
Mackerel	Pinto beans	Sea Bass	Lemon
Sardines	Millet	Trout	Nutmeg
Sole	Brown Rice	Soybean	Black pepper
Navy bean	Bay leaf	Wild rice	Safflower
Lentil	Dill	Unsalted butter	Quinoa
Basil	Ginger	Kelp	
Cayenne	White pepper	Mustard seeds	
Garlic	Sesame	Paprika	
Lime	Amaranth	Poppy Seed	
Olive Oil		Thyme	
Pepper		Gooseberries	
Chili			

6. Examples of Daily Menus

-1-

Breakfast	Two ricecakes spread with cashew butter
Lunch	Broiled chicken with lemon and veggies
Snack	Three small packages of corn chips
Dinner	Two ricecakes spread with cashew butter
Snack	Hand full of raw cashews

Drink Tea and Water

-2-

Breakfast	1/2 mango and kiwi
Lunch	Veal chop sauteed in butter Steamed 1/2 corn cob, beet, carrot, asparagus
Snack	Large package of "health" corn chips
Dinner	Scampi sauteed in butter and garlic Steamed green beans, acorn squash and two slices of yams

Water and Tea (Pau D'Arco)

-3-

Breakfast	1/2 mango and 1/2 banana
Snack	1 ricecake spread with cashew butter
Lunch	2 large bowls homemade lentil soup (onion, carrot, chinese chard, chicken leg, garlic and lentils) Boiled artichoke
Dinner	Chicken leg broiled with water mixture and steamed vegetables
Snack	Pumpkin seeds and raw cashews

52

-4-

Breakfast   1 kiwi and 1 1/2 bananas

Lunch   Charcoal broiled red snapper
Steamed vegetables

Dinner   Lots of buckwheat
Steamed 1/2 cob corn, asparagus and 1/4 acorn
squash

Snack   Bowl of popcorn popped with air

-5-

Breakfast   1/4 honeydew melon

Lunch   Small piece of sturgeon sauteed with lime, dill
and pepper, steamed carrots and asparagus

Snack   2 ricecakes

Dinner   Tuna steak marinated with olive oil, dill and
garlic, baked potato with butter, salt and
pepper and corn on the cob

Snack   3 ricecakes

-6-

Breakfast   1 kiwi and 1/4 honeydew melon

Lunch   3 ricecakes, cold broiled salmon, corn chips

Snack   1 kiwi and 1/2 papaya

Dinner   1/2 skinny chicken, broiled with lemon
Brown and wild rice, steamed herbs and green
beans

-7-

Breakfast   1/4 honeydew
2 wild rice cakes

Lunch   1/2 broiled chicken
1 small yam
Green lettuce salad

Dinner	2 egg spinach omelette 2 c. buckwheat
Snack	2 ricecakes spread with butter

-8-

Breakfast	1/4 honeydew melon and 1/2 c. blueberries
Lunch	2 egg onion omelette, 3/4 c. brown rice and raw spinach salad with oil and lemon
Dinner	Stir fried turkey, onion and broccoli with brown rice

-9-

Breakfast	2 soft boiled eggs and 2 c. buckwheat
Snack	1 package corn chips
Lunch	Broiled tuna marinated in oil, lemon, basil Steamed beet greens and crookneck squash
Dinner	Poached salmon Steamed pea pods and green beans
Snack	2 ricecakes spread with almond butter

-10-

Breakfast	1/2 mango and 1 kiwi
Snack	1 small package corn chips
Lunch	2 broiled chicken thighs without skin and garlic Steamed beet, summer squash, acorn squash and beet greens
Dinner	Salade Mimosa - spinach and butter lettuce with 1 chopped egg and ricecake croutons. Dressing of garlic, lemon juice, olive oil, pepper
Snack	Handful of dry roasted cashews

-11-

Breakfast	1/2 mango, 1/8 honeydew and 1 kiwi
Lunch	Salmon steak, sauteed with butter, basil and garlic Steamed asparagus and pea pods
Snack	1 small bag each potato chips and corn chops, health variety
Dinner	Charcoal broiled catfish with brown rice
Snack	Buckwheat rice crackers

-12-

Breakfast	Quinoa cereal
Lunch	Green salad with lemon Boiled potatoes and broccoli Dry broiled salmon
Snack	1 ricecake with roasted almond butter Few ricechips
Dinner	Baked red snapper Zucchini sauteed with onion, garlic, cilantro and sunflower seeds in butter Brown rice
Snack	1 ricecake with cashew butter

-13-

Breakfast	1 papaya spritzed with lime juice
Snack	1 large package of corn chips
Lunch	Lentil soup
Dinner	1/2 broiled chicken Steamed acorn squash, asparagus, beet
Snack	Handful of raw cashews

-14-

Breakfast   2 ricecakes spread thin with cashew butter

Lunch   Red snapper, sauteed with butter, garlic and
                   basil
                   Steamed beet, acorn squash, pea pods, leek

Dinner   Baked potato with butter and pepper, stir fried
                   onion, asparagus and pea pods

Snack   Buckwheat and brown rice snaps

-15-

Breakfast   Honeydew (1/8), 1/2 small mango and few rasp-
                   berries

Lunch   1 large package corn chips

Dinner   1/2 broiled chicken with lemon
                   Romaine lettuce and dressing
                   Baked potato with butter

-16-

Breakfast   Quinoa cereal

Lunch   Small piece of sturgeon sauteed in butter
                   Corn from corn on the cob and one beet, steamed

Snack   Two small packages corn chips

Dinner   Stir fried bok choy, onion and broccoli and rice

Snack   Handful of sunflower seeds and raw almonds

-17-

Breakfast   Squash blossom 2 egg omelette

Lunch   Romaine salad with oil and lemon juice dressing
                   1/2 Shelton chicken broiled

Dinner   2 packages health crackers and 1 package (small)
                   corn chips followed later by 1 ricecake spread
                   very thinly with cashew butter

-18-

Breakfast   Cooked brown rice cereal made with water

Snack   Almonds, raw and unsalted

Lunch   3 oz. sturgeon sauteed in butter and fresh dill
             with spinach salad - olive oil and lemon
             dressing

Dinner   4 beef ribs (not meaty and not particularly
             fatty)
             Baked potato and 1 1/2 baby eggplants sauteed in
             garlic basil and olive oil

-19-

Breakfast   One banana

Snack   Raw cashew nuts and sesame seeds

Lunch   Bay scallops, sauteed with pine nuts and chives
             in butter
             Steamed mixed veggies

-20-

Breakfast   1/2 papaya

Lunch   1/2 broiled chicken, briefly marinated in lemon,
             ginger and olive oil
             Steamed beet, yellow squash

Dinner   Corn on the cob, 1 crookneck squash, 5 tiny
             carrots steamed, brown rice

-21-

Breakfast   1/2 papaya and 1 banana

Lunch   Tuna sauteed in butter and raw spinach salad
             with garlic, olive oil and lemon juice

Snack   Small package corn tortilla chips without salt

Dinner   Broiled catfish, buttered carrots and red
             potatoes

57

-22-

Breakfast	1/4 papaya and some strawberries
Snack	Mixture of cashews and almonds
Lunch	Orange roughy and green salad with garlic, oil and lemon
Dinner	Sturgeon, sauteed in butter Corn on the cob
Snack	Corn chips

-23-

Breakfast	Small piece pink honeydew melon 1 banana
Lunch	3 ricecakes with cashew butter
Dinner	1/2 duckling roti with baked potato and steamed zucchini
Snack	Popcorn
Drinks	Water and tea (Pau D'Arco)

7. Dietary Food Suggestions

Chew food thoroughly 20 times each mouthful. Digestion begins in the mouth with the enzymes in your saliva.

Drink liquids between meals, NOT WITH MEALS, because the liquids will dilute the digestive juices.

Eat less and chew well when emotionally upset since the digestive chemistry is changed, preventing a complete digestion.

Avoid overcooking since vitamins, enzymes and protein are all heat sensitive.

It is best to eat small portions more often than large portions less often, since the Spleen will digest smaller amounts more easily.

Avoid foods to which you are allergic; at the same time, avoid eating and drinking the same thing two days in a row. Exceptions are brown rice and water.

Avoid distractions while eating such as TV, radio, reading or driving, since you will not focus on thoroughly chewing and maintaining a relaxed, enjoyable mental state which assists digestion and assimilation.

Read labels and ingredients on boxed, canned and packaged foods. When dining out, question your server as to the ingredients used in the food you are ordering. Especially for the Candida patient, it is important to know what he eats.

Keep a brief food-symptom-feeling journal of everything you eat or drink to learn more about foods and how they affect your health. Record them over a period of time and review the records.

Do not eat protein with starches and fruits. Also, avoid any kind of fruit with starch. Ideally, eat the tropical fruits by themselves, as a breakfast. Do not combine honeydew melon (or other melons) with any other food.

Your willingness to improve the quality of your life through healthier food choices and meal planning is a very significant step toward better health. Your willingness and action will produce the desired result. Following a healthy diet will make you more aware of the "garbage" people eat. You will be stimulated to do better and acquire the energy, the body, health, mental and physical powers, that you always dreamed of.

The area of greatest misunderstanding and confusion in the field of nutrition is **the failure to properly understand and interpret the symptoms and changes that follow the beginning of a better nutritional program.** When we introduce foods of higher quality in place of lower quality ones, we have to understand the sudden onset of new, and not always, improved symptoms.

This is exactly what happens to the Candida patient when s/he switches from the regular junk food or food rich in yeast, to a protein-rich quality diet. The closer the food will come to the natural state in which it occurs, the higher the quality. Nuts and seeds, eaten in their natural state (unsalted and raw), are superior to chicken which, in its turn, is superior to beef. The quality of a nutritional program is also improved by omitting toxic substances such as coffee, tea, chocolate, tobacco, salt, etc.

A few important rules have to be taken into consideration by the patient who wants to recover from illness through a high quality diet. There is no doubt: the HIGHER the quality of food we eat, the QUICKER we recover from disease, provided, of course, we are able to properly digest and assimilate. Proper food combining, proper order of eating the different kinds of food (the most easily digested food first), consuming the correct quantity and the correct time of eating (when hungry and not by the clock), are corner-stones in our eating habits.

Following these rules should give us joy, a state of well-being and relaxation? Not quite. At least not immediately. The body still has to discard lower-grade materials and make room for these improved superior ones. Every cell in our body has amazing intelligence and aims always for improvement for better health, even though we do mostly all we can to interfere with this process.

What are the signs that become evident when we first omit the lower-grade foods and instead, introduce superior foods? Toxic stimulants and lower-quality foods, where salt and spices have been added, have one thing in common: they are more stimulating than nut and vegetable proteins. Consequently, there will be a slower heart rate and initial letdown that lasts about 10 days and is followed by an increase in strength; this initial period is the **regeneration period.** Many patients stop their diet during this phase, "feeling better on the junk diet - the new one making them feeling weak." In this regeneration phase, there is a shunting of energy from the exterior to the interior, or from the skin and muscles to the internal organs. Of course, this temporary muscle weakness is felt as a decrease in energy, since all the energy available is required to build up or balance out the internal organs. In this crucial phase, it is very clear that the patient will have to rest more and restrict manual labor and sport activities. Many Candida patients will experience this already in the first week of the diet; many cannot stay on their jobs and take a leave of absence. Success in recovery of health hinges upon the correct understanding of this point-realizing that the body is using its main energies in the most important internal work. So please, just coast in your social obligations until you are out of the woods.

As the food quality is raised, interesting symptoms start to appear. The body starts to remove all the garbage, all the gross body obstructions. Wastes are certainly more rapidly discarded, then new tissue is made from the new, improved food. This becomes evident as weight loss. This is very clear in the case of the Candida patient: if he follows the anti-yeast diet well, s/he has to loose weight. Lack of weight loss is either due to non-compliance with the diet or bad elimination of the garbage deposited in the tissues. Some patients are worried because of the continuous weight loss (although most are elated to finally lose some weight), but mostly, this phase is followed by a **stabilization**. Here, the weight remains stable; discarded material is equal to the amount of tissue formed by the more vital food.

Finally, due to the improved absorption and assimilation, there will be an **ANABOLIC** stage with minimal weight gain and increased energy.

One of the symptoms that occur on a cleansing diet, such as the anti-Candida one, upsets most of my female patients. Often, there are skin eruptions and boils, especially on the face. Failure of understanding this symptom, leads to a catastrophe. Lots of doctors will diagnose these skin rashes as allergies, prescribing the devil's advocate, a cortisone unguent. They do not understand that this process is a favorable prognosis, well-known in acupuncture: we bring the toxins from the interior to the exterior. Discarding these toxins are saving you from more serious diseases, especially degenerative ones. Often, the Candida patient has "colds," with coughing up phlegm and even low-grade fevers. The biggest mistake we can do is try to stop these symptoms with medications, since they are part of a curing process. It is obvious at this point that patients who had junk diets for most of their lives, will manifest more of these unpleasant, but temporary, symptoms than people who have eaten better foods throughout their lives. So be happy when you observe these signs and realize that your body becomes healthier with the day. Visualize this whole process as waste leaving your body, therefore, unable to bring further pain and havoc.

Some patients also believe that once they are in the upgrade scale, perfection or the golden medal is just around the corner. Alas, health returns in cycles; after a better diet, you have alternating great days but also, shorter times of negative symptoms. Also, do not forget that following a "clean" diet will make you more sensitive to garbage food.

Before, you felt lousy all the time. Now that you reached peak energy, sugar, for instance, will crush you and wipe you out for a day. Be glad your body does not allow you to eat inferior food anymore. Nature has given you a second chance through purer diet and natural foods. Sit back and enjoy what happens: you can experience what it really is to feel healthy and fully alive!

B. KILL THE CANDIDA

After being the victims of medications for such a long time, most patients are not very enthusiastic about returning to any medication at all. This is understandable. However, as I already stressed before, as an enemy, Candida is a tough one! It took clever advantage of your weakened immune system in order to invade your body. In their turn, the yeast cells will continue to suppress your very important defense mechanisms. And this is where the anti-yeast medication comes into play: its role is to break this vicious cycle. But it is important to realize that medication intake alone will not do the job. This part of the treatment is the easiest: we already live in a world sensitized to medication intake. Again, we have to stress the importance of all the steps of the treatment. The different anti-yeast medications are described in chronological order, with their advantages and disadvantages.

1. NYSTATIN POWDER

Numerous cases document the efficacy of the initial drug of choice, Nystatin, in treating the atypical Candida patient. A very small dose is taken in the beginning (the tip of a toothpick), and every day the dose is built up when tolerated.

Day 1: one toothpick
Day 2: two toothpicks
Day 3: three toothpicks when tolerated
Day 4: 1/8 tsp. and 2 toothpicks
Day 5: twice a 1/8 tsp. and 1 toothpick
Day 6: three times a 1/8 tsp.
Day 7: 1/4 tsp. and 1/8 tsp. bid
Day 8: 1/4 tsp. bid and 1/8 tsp. once a day
Day 9: 1/4 tsp. tid

The dose is built up to sometimes a full teaspoon three times a day when the patient tolerates it.

What are the advantages?

Mixed in some water, it is easy to take. It will also dissolve rather easily in water to add to a small enema, in this way reaching the sigmoid and the rectum in high concentration. In case of postnasal drip, the powder is very useful to sniff, bringing a high concentration of the drug in the nasal cavity, fertile ground for Candida.

Disadvantages?

They are rather numerous. First, it is rather expensive and very few pharmacies carry it. A major disadvantage is that Nystatin is NOT A BROAD SPECTRUM fungicide. While effective for certain strains of Candida, numerous, potentially pathogenic fungi are unaffected by it. Strains of Candida resistant to Nystatin have been described. It is not unreasonable to assume that as with antibacterial antibiotics, an increased use of Nystatin will induce the emergence of Nystatin resistant strains.

Nystatin is a mold by-product and may cause allergic reactions in the mold-sensitive patient. In my practice, up to fifty percent of the patients had this problem. It is also difficult to determine the proper individual dose: this is different from person to person, and it is hard for the patient to distinguish adverse reactions from die-off symptoms. Some adverse reactions are nausea and vomiting, while withdrawal symptoms are usually noted when the Nystatin intake in halted. This is nothing unusual, as I have seen patients who were on Nystatin intake for several years! In the generic sense, Nystatin is a potent antibiotic and the long term effects of its use on normal bacterial and normal fungal intestinal flora are not clear.

These negative characteristics of Nystatin suggest the need for other agents which alone or synergistically minimize the drawbacks, while maintaining or exceeding Nystatin's record of safety and efficacy.

In practice, I never would prescribe it as a first line medication, but keep it in mind for resistant cases and local use.

2.   NIZAROL TABLETS, 200 mg.

This is a very potent antifungal drug. It is a synthetic BROAD SPECTRUM antifungal agent available in white tablets, each containing 200 mg ketoconazole.

It is THE antifungal medication for the presence of Candida in the esophagus. Patients with burning in the chest, and difficulties to swallow should add this drug to their therapeutic regimen. Nizarol requires acidity for dissolution. If concomitant antacids or Tagamet (H2 blocker) are needed, they should be given at least two hours after Nizarol administration. This medication is contraindicated in case of pregnancy and breast feeding.

Nizarol is usually well tolerated. The most frequent adverse reactions are nausea and vomiting, which occur only in 3% of the patients. In infrequent cases, liver damage has been noticed. Therefore, a liver blood test is done before each onset of this medication. After one month of treatment, the test is repeated.

Nizarol is easy to take since it only requires one tablet daily. I like to prescribe it in the above-mentioned cases and together with other anti-fungal medications to avoid resistance for some organisms.

3.   FUNGIZONE TABLETS, 100 mg an 250 mg

Unfortunately, this medication is not yet approved by the FDA. Although it has been used in Europe for at least fifteen years with NO adverse reactions, the FDA never okayed the medication in the form of TABLETS. Strangely enough, the IV form of this same medication has been approved. Strangely, because in this form it is very toxic, so toxic that it can only be administered in a hospital. It is harmful to the kidneys while a variety of other side effects have been noted. In this country, the ointment and cream are also approved.

I have prescribed it many times in Europe (tablet form) without noticing any side effect at all. It is definitely a broad spectrum anti-fungal medication, superior to the Nystatin. The only possible side effect was sometimes a prolonging in the menstrual cycle, returning to normal after interrupting the medication.

The usual dose is 1000 mgs. daily, spread over the day. The 250 mg. tablet is easy to obtain in France, where not even a prescription is needed. This way, many patients obtained the medication when they were vacationing in Europe.

It is important to notice that intake of laxativa and psyllium will aggravate the Candida symptoms. In case of constipation, other measurements as noted in C (page # 80) are taken.

4. CAPRYSTATIN

Caprystatin contains 100 mgs. of Caprycillic acid. Already as far back as 1954, the effectiveness of this medication in vitro studies was demonstrated. It was with surprise that patients and doctors who expected enormous benefits from this product, noted that the medication had disappointing results to say the least. Further studies have improved the quality and now it is certainly a possibility in the treatment of Candidiasis.

Caprystatin is administered at least one hour before or after meals. If gastrointestinal discomfort is noted, it may be taken with meals.

What is the dose?

First week, one tablet, two times daily. The second week, two tablets twice daily, following by three tablets daily. The maintenance dose is two tablets daily. Average duration of treatment with Caprystatin is 2-3 months at a therapeutic dose, followed by 4-6 months as a maintenance dose. This is due to the fact that it contains only 100 mgs of Caprycillic acid, a sharp contrast with the later medications, containing 300 mgs Caprycillic acid in each tablet. Then again, it might be an advantage for highly allergic patients and patients who suffer too much from die-off symptoms!

Caprystatin is not advised in pregnancy and in patients with a history of fiber intolerance (it contains a high amount of fiber!)

What is the action of Caprystatin against Candida?

Fatty acid production by indigenous bacteria is a major factor in maintaining a balanced intestinal microflora. Caprycillic acid is a fatty acid, increasing the amount of fatty acid production in case of disruption by antibiotica and immunosuppressive drugs.

5. TANALBIT tablets

It contains 550 mg of Zinc-Salicylo-Tannate, an anti-fungal preparation. It is not a first-line drug such as the Caprycillic acid preparations, but it is certainly a valid alternative for people who cannot handle the die-off symptoms.

The regular dose is 2 and 2 tablets daily, for fourteen days. After an interruption of 2 weeks, another 2 weeks of medication is taken. This cycle is continued till complete cure has been obtained. No known side-effects.

6. CAPRYLLIN Tablets (GRL)

Scientific literature has long indicated that Caprycillic acid should be effective in killing Candida Albicans. However, the caprycillic acid products available until recently have yielded very disappointing results. Therefore, further studies with caprycillic acid were done and renewed. Very effective medications were brought on the market under different names (Capricin, Capryllin, ...) but, we mention Capryllin since it has all the advantages of the other products, but a lower price.

The active agent is also the caprycillic agent, but this time it is formulated as a time release preparation. The coating of Capryllin allows for slow uniform release of

Caprycillic acid along the entire length of the gastrointestinal tract. What is the dose?

It has been determined with stool cultures that a dosage of twelve capsules divided in three or two doses over the day, will eliminate almost all of the Candida, if Capryllin was taken for 16 days. Afterwards, a maintenance dose of two tablets, twice a day for a couple of months, will avoid relapses. It is important during that time to try to build up the immune system so that recurrences will not happen.

Practically, I like to start the dosage with 1 capsule three times a day for one day. The second day, 2 capsules tid, the third day 3 capsules tid and the fourth day on till the sixteenth, 4 capsules, three times a day. This way the patient's body adjusts to the die-off symptoms. We may not forget that up till they come in for therapy, the patient's diet was loaded with yeast. If together with the anti-yeast diet, the lactobacillus, garlic and Pau D'Arco tea, an anti-fungal medication is taken from the first day of treatment on, the die-off will be too severe, causing the patient to cease any therapy. More about this at the end of this chapter (page # 74).

It is advised to take the capsules with food, since some nausea or burping up of a soapy taste can occur if taken on an empty stomach.

The major advantages of Capryllin, such as its low price, its time released effect and the 300 mgs of Caprycillic acid it contains, makes Capryllin the first drug choice at this moment.

7.   KANTITA

Its ingredients list three herbs: Red Clover, Yellow Dock and Condurango. The normal dosage is 2 capsules, 3 times daily. This product is excellent to start with extremely sensitive patients. It is well tolerated and it has a mild killing effect. But even with this product, sensitivity and allergy can appear.

The Yellow Dock Root used in this preparation has as nutrients, vitamins A, C, Manganese, Nickel and Iron. It's medicinal use is that of a blood builder, astringent, cholagogue and laxative. It is respected as a nutritive tonic. It is available in health food stores.

8.   YEAST FIGHTERS

These yeast fighters are taken in a dose of 5 capsules daily. They contain Lactobacillus Ac. 1000 mgs (2.5 billions), natural caprycillic acid 100 mgs, Biotin 900 mcg. and Fiber blend 3500 mgs. This product is certainly a solution for the first week of therapy and as an adjuvant with very sensitive patients. The high fiber content is helpful in the constipation.

9.   CANDIDA CLEANSE

It claims to provide the most potent antifungal herbs in the world. It also includes other botanicals whose properties are noted for their abilities to strengthen the digestive tract, the immune system and the metabolic system. It includes in each tablet active cells of acidophilus, bulgaricus and bifidus. These cultures are from carrot powder. It contains Black Walnut concentrate, Pau D'Arco powder, Radix Astragalus, Biotin, Spirulina and Acidophilus to name a few of its substances. The suggested dosis is 2 tablets daily, between meals during the first two weeks, three tablets the third and fourth weeks; one tablet thereafter.

A disadvantage is the small concentration of Acidophilus. It is my belief that this dosage is not enough to replace the normal flora. Advantages are the 50 mcgs of Biotin, the spirulina and the black walnut concentrate, efficient against worms and parasites.

10.   GARLIC

The world has always been divided in two camps: those who love garlic and those who detest it. The first camp would include the Egyptian pharaohs who were entombed with clay and wood carvings of garlic and onions to ensure that meals in afterlife would be well seasoned. It would include the Jews who wandered for many years in the Sinai wilderness, fondly remembering "the fish we eat in Egypt so freely, and the leeks, onions and garlic."

The camp of the onion and garlic haters would include the ancient Greeks, who considered the odor of garlic and onion eaters vulgar, and the Egyptian priests who "kept themselves clear from it..."

Chemists must be included among the garlic lovers. For them, the reasons are professional. In recent times, clinical experiments have confirmed most of those ancient ideas about garlic powder. In fact, it appears that the healing powers of garlic may be far greater than previously anticipated.

Garlic has been on the breath of the physically fit and the widely avoided for over 5000 years and is now being rediscovered all over again by the medical and scientific community. Garlic has a long history of medicinal uses. The Babylonians used it to treat disease as early as 3000 B.C. In Egypt, the Pharaohs were entombed with clay and wood carvings of garlic to ensure that meals in the afterworld would be well-seasoned. Garlic was the food of the slaves working on the Pyramids to give them strength to endure hard labor. The Greek athletes took garlic (not steroids) for increased energy and stamina.

The Romans used it as a diuretic and worm expeller. Aristophanes believed that garlic juice could restore man's flagging virility. Hippocrates, the father of medicine, used garlic for a wide variety of ailments. Louis Pasteur, the great microbiologist, was a firm believer in garlic because of its anti-microbial and anti-bacterial activity. Albert Schweitzer used garlic in Africa for the treatment of dysentery and cholera.

Garlic was used as an antiseptic for the prevention of gangrene and septic poisoning during World Wars I and II and saved thousands and thousands of lives. The Soviet government has imported garlic from Europe to fight flu epidemic, at one time importing 500 tons of garlic for their population. At the turn of the last century, American family doctors treated asthma, whooping cough, and tuberculosis with garlic and had excellent results. Garlic has been effective against several of the bacteria cultures, resistent to commonly used antibiotics including penicillin, various tetracyclines, and streptomycin. Attention to anti-fungal powers was established when sufferers of fungus-caused inflammation of the brain, cryptococcal meningitis, were treated with garlic. Garlic along, or garlic with other drugs, was 85% effective. Garlic extract was more effective than nystatin against pathogenic yeast, especially C. albican.[1]

Moses A. Adetumbia, Ph. D, from Loma Linda University, School of Medicine, demonstrated how garlic extract inhibited the growth of Candida in an experiment described in his paper "Anti-Candida Activity of Garlic." Garlic killed the yeast with its sulfur containing anti-fungal and anti-microbial compounds. Dr. Benjamin Lau, M.D., Ph. D., conducts research studies on natural products in health at Loma Linda University. This university's influence in the health field is worldwide. Dr. Lau has reviewed garlic and especially a deoxidized - deodorized garlic extract, **KYOLIC**, on human health in a series of articles in journals such as "Medical Hypothesis" and "Nutrition Research." Dr. Lau points out that raw garlic may produce heartburn, diarrhea, and anemia but these problems do not occur with KYOLIC, an organically grown and biologically active garlic, aged without the use of heat. He also reviewed the tendency of the extract to reduce thrombotic accidents in which clots may precipitate coronary attacks, strokes, and phlebitis.

[1] Moore-Atkins, School of Health Science, University of Massachusetts.

Three major constituents in raw garlic, including S-allyl cysteine, gave protection to liver cells and against carbon tetrachloride poisoning. This is the subject of a patent application by **WAKUNAGA PHARMACEUTICAL** (makers of KYOLIC). Dr. Lau has performed experiments on increased physical endurance of the heart brought about by the adminstration of KYOLIC. KYOLIC has been shown to be effective in controlling vaginitis, caused by Candida albicans, and through a chemical complexing reaction with foreign proteins to help in preventing viral infections.

KYOLIC is one of the best natural sources of Germanium, a potential agent in the treatment of cancer. Dr. Lau and several urologists used liquid KYOLIC, odorless garlic, as a non-specific immune stimulant in bladder cancer in mice. It appears that the sulfhydrol compounds (SH group) in KYOLIC inhibited the growth of bladder cancer without side effects. Two internists working with Dr. Lau showed how KYOLIC lowered cholesterol and triglycerides and elevated the good guys, the HDL (high density lipoproteins). It is the HDL that promotes the removal of cholesterol from the artery walls. In people 50 and over, the HDL measurement is the best single lab test to predict not only the occurrence of coronary artery disease but survival itself. One of Dr. Lau's students showed garlic extract inhibited the growth of coccidiodes immitis (cause of Valley Fever), a common disease in California. Dr. Norton Lugar, one of the most respected medical doctors, wrote recently on garlic lowering high blood pressure, "For those who find the odor of garlic offensive, KYOLIC, an aged deodorized garlic, retains the therapeutic effects of raw garlic without the odor." KYOLIC's selenium content is the highest in garlic products and selenium apparently stimulates the body's immune response mechanism. KYOLIC retains the highest amount of allicin (Nature's antibiotic). KYOLIC is the only garlic product produced in a GMP factory. It is checked 250 times during production, and supported by GLP (Good Laboratory Practice). KYOLIC is the only garlic

product given toxicity tests and clinical tests. The twenty
month natural aging process makes its stable, predigested,
and free of any known side effects.

A nationally televised documentary on Candida is in the
making, and will feature patients who suffered from Candida
albicans along with severe chemical sensitivities who
completely overcame their conditions with daily use of KYOLIC
and a nutritious diet.

American medicine is just now catching up with research
into garlic remedies. Scientific medicine will have to
practice a little humility, after all...garlic could not be
deceiving people for all those centuries.

KYOLIC INFO UPDATE...

Editorials, testimonials, and interesting newsbits have
been cropping up recently involving Kyolic. Here is an
update...

1. KYOLIC is listed in the PDR (Physicians' Desk Reference for (Non-Prescription Drugs".) This extremely important
reference book is used by 300,000 medical practitioners.

2. 1982 issue of "The Journal of Indiana State Medical
Assn." "A Japanese-developed garlic extract called Kyolic is
recommended for preventing heart disease and arteriosclero-
sis, for maintaining cholesterol levels in normal range and
for improving the body's immune system. The extract is
enclosed in a capsule and reportedly does not cause
unpleasant side effects. Added benefits are the lowering of
blood sugar in diabetes and the raising of blood sugar in
hypoglycemia."

3. 1984 issue of "The U.S. Navy Reserve Medical Center"
publication - "Garlic and onions contain anti-coagulant
substances that may prevent heart attacks. They have a
tendency to thin the blood, thus preventing blood clots."

4. "The Merck Index," 9th edition - Allicin, the anti-
bacterial principal of garlic was isolated by scientists in
1944. Allicin is still listed under "Therapeutic category"
as an anti-microbial in the Merck Index, a nationally

respected encyclopedia of chemicals and drugs.

5. Wakunaga Pharmaceutical Co., makers of Kyolic, was the only garlic producer invited to the World Health Organization Conference on Herbs, in 1982, where they presented conclusive clinical studies on the effectiveness of their garlic preparation.

11. PAU D'ARCO TEA

Quickly gaining popularity is the South American herb Pau D'Arco, which is often referred to by its other Spanish names: Ipe Roxa, Lapacho and Taheebo. It is currently hailed for its effects on cancer (in South America) and Candida.

Pau D'Arco is the inner bark of a large tree that flowers a vibrant pink, purple or yellow, depending on the species. Throughout South America, Pau D'Arco is used as a remedy for immune system-related problems, such as colds, fevers, infections, snake bites. It was one of the major healing herbs used by the Incas.

Toxicity of Pau D'Arco is very low. It may loosen the bowels, which is frequently desirable in the Candida patient. It is available as a tea, in tea bags, but capsules are also on the market. Up to three - four cups a day may be taken, while it is an excellent idea to use some of the tea together with Lactobacillus in an enema. Using an enema twice a week quickly brings relief of some of the die-off symptoms, especially brainfog.

As you can see, we already made quite a progress, but, hopefully, this is not the end. Still too many patients cannot take any of the above medications because they are "allergic" to anything. And in about 50% of the patients, there will be a die-off phenomenon.

WHAT IS THIS DIE-OFF PHENOMENON?

Especially with high doses of Caprycillic acid, all of a sudden thousands of yeast cells will be killed. The dead toxins formed from these yeast cells will overwhelm the patient's organism, causing symptoms sometimes more uncomfortable than the symptoms of the disease itself. "I am not better, but worse" is a frequently heard complaint in the beginning of the therapy. These die-off symptoms usually appear between the 2nd and 5th day of medication intake and will usually last for one week (sometimes even two). After this period most of the candida cells are dead and eliminated, so that less and less cells have to be killed, limiting the amount of the die-off.

WHAT ARE THE SYMPTOMS?

Any of the yeast connected symptoms may appear, but especially flu-like symptoms, brain symptoms such as "foggy thinking," concentration and memory decrease, muscle and joint pains, tightness in the chest with palpitations and even a feeling of a film over the eyes with irritation will surface during the die-off. It is not unfamiliar that the patient states that he feels drunk, putting him in a state of incapacity. Thinking about these symptoms, it is no wonder that almost 50% of the Candida patients have been admitted in a psychiatric ward with all the disastrous consequences.

HOW DO WE AVOID OR ALLEVIATE THE DIE-OFF SYMPTOMS?

. Follow the anti-yeast diet as strictly as possible, especially during the first two weeks on anti-yeast medication (in case of Capryllin); each time you cheat, you give the yeast cells a chance to grow.

. Start taking the anti-yeast medication the second week after your first visit to the doctor; the first week you will start with the diet, acupuncture, supplements (Acidophilus) and natural killers such as garlic and Pau D'Arco tea. The latter ones will already kill a lot of yeast cells, clearing the way for Capryllin to do the definite kill.

. Do not start with the full dose of the medication but rather build the medication up so that your body can adjust to the die-off.

. If possible, take vacation during the period you expect the heaviest die-off, or plan it during the weekend.

. When having foggy brain symptoms, drink a lot of water with lemon juice, it will clear toxins.

. Make sure you have regular bowel movements; via the stool you eliminate toxins; see C (Evaluation of Toxines).

. Use the brushing technique: take a regular clothes brush and brush as if you were cleaning your clothes. Brush the following area: starting at the lower inside of the leg, brush your way up to the groin; then brush downward starting with the upper lateral side of the thigh, all the way to the ankle; continue on the outer side of the arm up from the wrist to the shoulder and then back down from the inside of the axilla to the wrist. What you are accomplishing with this is stimulating all the meridians in the direction of the stream of energy, double-checking any stagnation and, therefore, eliminating toxins.

In spite of all this, still many patients go through very uncomfortable die-off symptoms, but once they go through it, the reward is great: it feels heavenly to be able to think straight for the first time in a long period, it gives the patient hope that there is a chance for improvement.

A very important reason for severe die-off symptoms, and cause for a foggy brain, is the occurrence of an "OPEN ILEO-CECAL valve." This valve is located at the junction of the small intestine (ileum) and the large intestine (first part or caecum). The function of this valve is to prevent the feces from backing up into the small intestine where it would be absorbed in the blood stream, poisoning the organism. A barium enema for X-rays will show this, but thanks to applied kinesiology, it is very simple to demonstrate that in almost 100% of Candida patients, this valve stays open permanently.

Patients killing the yeast cells with the anti-fungal therapy, garlic, Pau D'Arco tea, etc. will set off a lot of toxins which will get through the open valve, and back up the whole gastrointestinal tract. Via absorption in the blood, they will cause the fogginess in the brain.

How do we recognize this open valve?

This is easily done with applied kinesiology: touching the area over the ileocecal valve (located slightly above the appendix) will produce weakness if the valve is open. The test is most accurate if the tested person wears a white cotton gown to neutralize the effect of the other clothes he is wearing.

How do we close the open Ileo-Cecal valve?

Your acupuncturist can close this valve readily by puncturing four points. What is even more important, the patient can do it himself by rubbing or massaging those same points.

Point 1: Spleen 1 point, located at the inside of the big toe. The point is easily located by drawing two lines next and under the nail. It will be located at the crossing of both lines. Rub the point on both feet.

Point 2: Large Intestine 3 point, located on the proximal side of the knuckle of the index finger. To be done on both hands.

Point 3: Bladder 58 point, located by placing 9 fingers next to each other, starting from the malleolus (external). The point is located on the line drawn from the mid-point of a line drawn between achilles tendon and Malleolus externus.

Point 4: Touch (not rubbing) the Bladder 58 point on the LEFT leg, while at the same time touching the Kidney point, number 7, on the RIGHT leg. Kidney 7 is located 3 fingers above the internal malleolus, on a line drawn from the midline on the line, connecting the malleolus internus with the Achilles tendon.

The result will be immediate as can be tested by the patient: as were before, there was an extreme weakness when touching the area of the value, this weakness will totally disappear! The patient can test himself to see how long the valve will stay closed. Repeat the procedure if necessary and eventually this valve will remain closed when the patient is totally balanced. The points are rubbed for about 15 seconds. Usually, this valve stays closed for about 14 days. Very weak patients might check it daily since there will be a tendency for it to open in the beginning.

One of my patients who is much in touch with her body described this closing of the valve while she was undergoing the acupuncture treatment: "I felt coolness, like my body temperature dropped five degrees (in acupuncture, a toxic syndrome is known as a "hot syndrome"). There was some release of energy, like an engine revived and ready to go; then, this subsided and I felt a muscle movement in the area of the ileo-cecal valve as though it was closing shut; then my head cleared."

Sometimes the clearing of the fogginess will not happen right a way, but a day later. The day of the treatment the patient has a strange, unfamiliar feeling, not painful nor uncomfortable: evidently, the valve may have been open for a long time.

C. EVACUATE TOXINS

One of the pillars in the success therapy of Candida is the maintaining of a regular bowel movement. Constipation is almost always present in the case of Candida, inducing die-off symptoms. We frequently see a "roller-coaster" phenomena: the patient feels excellent at 9 o'clock in the morning, two hours later, unexpectedly, he feels 180 degrees different. This is due to the presence of toxins: at nine in the morning this patient's colon was relatively free of toxins, but after breakfast and the first dosage of medication, yeast cells are killed and form toxins. If the patient does not evacuate these toxins immediately, he will be overwhelmed. These sudden changes in behavior do not always contribute to the acceptance of the disease by family members or friends.

I cannot list all the possible and natural remedies that are available to ensure a normal stool. But, I list here the ones that have proven to be effective in my practice.

1. FIBERS IN DIET

Dietary fiber is a broad term covering a complex mixture of many substances. Initially, it was defined as being the roughage of plants left after the digestive process. Grain fibers such as wheat or rice bran are largely insoluble. By absorbing water and swelling within the intestines, they tend to reduce the bowel transit time between intake and elimination.

Recently, crude fibers include some substances such as pectins, gums and mucilages found in many fruits. They form viscous solutions that soften the stool and may prolong the nutrient transport time in the gastrointestinal tract.

Fiber is not absorbed by the body and thus is not defined as one of the essential nutrients. There are no minimum daily requirements set for it as there are for various vitamins and minerals.

Scientists became aware of the crucial role of fiber in the diet through studies of native Japanese who, upon arriving in Hawaii, adopted the low fiber, high fat Western Diet. They suddenly developed heart and intestinal diseases previously unknown to them, including appendicitis, diverticulitis, cancer of the colon, diabetes, myocardial infarction and obesity.

A key factor in the high-fiber diet is rapid transit time from intake to elimination. Studies have shown that African children on their native diet have transit times of eight to twelve hours, while elderly Britons may have transit times of up to fourteen DAYS! The stool made softer and bulkier by pectins and grain, roughage is easier for the colon to move along, inhibits the excessive growth of bacteria and, by causing the colon to stretch to handle the increased bulk, permits relatively fewer carcinogens to come into contact with the walls of the intestines. In some people, fiber may also help to inhibit the absorption of cholesterol.

Adhering to a well-balanced, low fat, high fiber diet makes it easier to lose weight since the greater bulkiness of high fiber foods causes most people to feel full and, thus, reduce their intake. And, of course, such a diet is usually low in calories.

Americans have diets that are abnormally low in fiber. We should increase our intake to 30 grams of fiber a day, depending on our size (larger individuals should consume more). However, do not add too much fiber at once: it takes a few days for the system to adjust. In some people too much fiber can cause gas, intestinal discomfort and loose stools, symptoms that are already present in most Candida patients. Also, be sure to increase your intake of water - six glasses a day - as an increase in fiber causes you to need more water in order to bulk up the stool. Also, be aware of the higher loss of trace elements and other important substances such as calcium, iron, zinc and magnesium. All of the latter elements are extremely important for the Candida patient:

either he has a deficiency of those or a deficiency will trigger or maintain the Candida growth.

You can easily add fiber to your diet by increasing the amount of fruits, vegetables and nuts that you serve. Perhaps one of the easiest meals at which to increase fiber is breakfast. Rice bran, nuts and brown rice should be among the favorite breakfasts for Candida patients.

2. COLON THERAPY AND ENEMAS

"Cleanse the bowel" has been a motto of any health-oriented doctor. The large intestine plays a major role in a wide range of diseases. When properly used, it is a lot more than just a simple lavage. It will include the analysis of the stool (in the case of the Candida patient, green mucosy stool is eliminated), and the irrigation of the colon with various solutions such as Pau D'Arco tea, Lactobacillus solutions and eventual low doses of anti-fungal medications. Our therapeutic goals are to re-balance the body chemistry, elimination of old impacted stool, and to bring a high concentration of anti-fungal substances to every corner of the colon.

Colonic therapy has fallen out of favor in recent times because it is more time consuming than the intake of laxatives. Again, we are victims of our lifestyle!

Indication for colonic therapy starts with recognition of the signs of colon imbalance. Watch out! Normal daily bowel movements do not rule out colon dysfunction. Despite enemas and laxatives, large amounts of impacted feces can be expelled through colonics.

The irrigation solutions are different from practitioner to practitioner. The most common solution is tap water, since it causes only mild inflammatory changes. Others use soapsuds or oil.

The therapist will frequently use supplemental Acidophilus and Pau D'Arco tea, for instance, to help establish the optimal pH and therapeutic milieu. This way we bring the highest concentration of the anti-fungal medication in places where oral therapy hardly reaches.

What are side effects of this colonic irrigation?

Transient symptoms of nausea and diarrhea, due to the increased reflux of bile in the stomach. There can be a potassium loss from tap water enemas, therefore, an intake of 20 mEq/L (1 capsule) daily will prevent a hypokalemia.

The apparatus should be easy to disinfect and it is even more practical to have the disposable tips (obturators). Modern machines use pressure gauges and automatic shut-off to ensure safety.

We can say that a colon cleansing is a gentle, warm water washing of the large intestine combined with some external massage. It is completely safe, beneficial and non-toxic. The procedure lasts about 45 minutes and is accomplished with an irrigation machine, utilizing pre-sterilized, disposable hoses and speculums. Since they are only used once, there is absolutely no danger of contamination.

The water dislodges toxic wastes in the colon which are then flushed out through the waste hose. A series of water filling and releases stimulates the expansion and contraction of the muscular walls. Combined with a changing of the water temperature from warm to cool. This exercises the colon and relieves the spasticity of it. How many Candida patients have come to me with the diagnosis of "Spastic Colon?" And, of course, even some colon X-rays were supporting this diagnosis. It might be magic to a gastroenterologist how a colon irrigation takes care of this "spasticity."

During the cleansing, most people are pleasantly surprised that they can relax during the entire procedure. Some patients think that colon irrigation might wash out the normal intestinal flora. First of all, a Candida patient has very little friendly bacteria left in his colon, and secondly, colon cleansings do NOT wash out flora. The colon irrigation on the other hand is an excellent opportunity to improve the bacterial balance in the colon by implanting

Acidophilus products.

Since colonic therapy will not cleanse the small intestines, the buildup there is eliminated with the help of Intestinal Cleaner and other nutritional aids (fresh vegetables and fruit juices).

What is the latest position of the AMA toward colonic therapy? In the public health letter of March '86, it is written:

"A recent Superior Court ruling has upheld the California Attorney General's opinion that performance of colonic irrigation constitutes the practice of medicine and that chiropractors, physical therapists and other non-physicians are precluded from performing this procedure.

Colonic irrigation, a series of enemas provided over a short time, generally through a gravity dependent apparatus, has been associated with transmission of enteric pathogens including Entamoeba and Shigella. Colonic irrigations can alter host defenses in otherwise healthy people and may cause injury to intestinal mucosa, removal of protective mucus and changes in bacterial flora which can facilitate disease when human pathogens are encountered.

Because of the proven hazards associated with colonic irrigation and the lack of any known benefits, the County of Los Angeles Department of Health Services and the State of California Department of Health Services recommend that no one, including physicians, should perform this procedure."

Enemas are also a must for most Candida patients. Take a baby enema, over the counter in most drug stores, and fill it with Acidophilus, Pau D'Arco tea and sometimes, with the anti-fungal medication you take. This way you get a high dosis of these yeast fighters in the more distal and high concentrated zones of Candida. The beneficial effect is almost immediately. It can be done even by the most emaciated patient. Two to three times weekly is a good average for any patient. It has shown especially to be of benefit in eliminating the fogginess of the brain.

3. SUPPLEMENTS

The yeast fighters are mentioned on page 69 . Another excellent product is CELGINATE (GRL). The tablet contains sea algae combined with celery root powder, making it an excellent bulking agent. It improves the bowel movement; the algae absorb many of the toxins, therefore, consumption of this product helps to clear the skin. Start with a dosis of three tablets with each meal and increase if possible to five tablets, tid. Celginate has been proven to give excellent results in the PMS syndrome and in the lowering of the blood cholesterol.

Amaranth, in the form of a cereal, is now produced by Arrowhead Mills, and is available in most health food stores. Considered an ideal breakfast, it will give the patient an ideal start in the morning.

4. OTHER METHODS

Adding a touch of lemon in water provides the patient with an ideal detoxification source. Drink up to eight glasses of water.

The brushing method is already mentioned on page   .

Acupuncture is a powerful weapon in maintaining a normal stool and evacuating the toxins. There are special points to be stimulated, located on the Large Intestine and Liver meridian.

An herbal medicine, Major Rhubarb, has been proven to be excellent for many patients. The bag comes with a little spoon: 3 little spoons in the evening ensures mostly a good BM. Other stimulant laxatives are: Aloe Vera, Cascara bark and Senna leaves/pods.

D. AVOID SPREADING TO THE BLOOD

We have discussed the spreading mechanism in Chapter V, page 21 . In order for the Candida patient to avoid the spreading to the bloodstream, and thus giving the opportunity to the yeast cells to invade almost all the organs, the interruption of the vicious cycle is a must and a priority! Biotin is the weapon in our hand. Biotin, taken in an amount of at least three MILLIGRAM, will cut the transformation cycle from the yeast to the fungus form. The daily dosis will be taken with the first dosis of the anti-fungal therapy. We may not forget that Biotin is a B-vitamin, feeding the fungus. However, the cutting of the vicious spreading cycle is more important.

The amount of the Biotin is important. Some patients come with their multivitamins to me indicating that there is some Biotin in it. However, this is always in a strength of MICRO-CENTIGRAM (mcg). This will not be enough for our purpose. The regular dosis will be 3-5 mg daily. Biotin has been administered to humans for prolonged periods with dosages as high as 40 mg/day without adverse effects. Biotin is one of the most active biological substances known; extremely small amounts have marked effects on the growth of a number of organisms. Biotin is one of many water soluble vitamins that stress can deplete. Biotin is essential in the conversion of carbohydrates to energy, and also plays a major role in the synthesis of fats and in protein metabolism. Other conditions known to be associated with lowered or deficient levels of Biotin are: loss of hair, anorexia, lassitude, muscle weakness, hypercholesterolemia and depression. The best available product on the market is the Biotin 5 mg tablet of GRL.

E. REPLACE THE INDIGENOUS (NATURALLY OCCURRING) FLORA

The composition of the normal gastrointestinal flora is discussed on page 21 . We already know that the presence of these billions of friendly bacteria (L. acidophilus and Bifidobacteria) are essential in order to inhibit the growth of yeast cells. Normal flora can be destroyed after only a few days of antibiotic use, for instance, and need to be replaced in order to avoid the creation of a favorable environment for the yeast. By supplementing your daily diet with stable, high potency L. acidophilus and Bifidobacteria, you are greatly enhancing your body's natural ability to keep dangerous and/or pathogenic microorganisms under control. As an added bonus, daily supplementation of Lactobacilli products increases the absorption of nutrients, reduces blood cholesterol levels, maximizes the efficiency of the digestive system, and greatly enhances the immune system.

ALLERGIES AND LACTOSE INTOLERANCE

There are many people that would benefit greatly from using L. acidophilus and Bifidobacteria supplements, but feel that they cannot successfully do so due to lactose intolerance or other milk-based allergies. They unwillingly purchase so-called "hypo-allergenic" (milk-free) products that claim to be superior in potency and viability due to the absence of milk in their processing methods. However, what the public is not aware of is the fact that by <u>not</u> culturing (or growing) their microorganisms in a milk base, the viability and potency are severely impaired. The most efficacious L. acidophilus and Bifidobacteria products currently on the market culture their microorganisms in a natural milk base because this is the most friendly and nurturing medium available. It is also the <u>only</u> medium in which the L. acidophilus is able to produce the natural antibiotic, <u>acidophilin</u>, which is one of the major benefits of acidophilus supplementation. In other words, the "hypo-allergenic" manufacturers are taking their microorganism out of their natural environment and placing them in hostile surroundings while making claims about increased benefits to the consumer, when in actuality, they are rendering these friendly bacteria virtually ineffective!

Also, it is now known that lactose-intolerant people do not manufacture "lactase," which is a naturally occurring enzyme whose function is to break down milk sugar into a more simple form which the body can then digest. The ingestion of even the slightest amount of milk products can cause extreme digestive disorders in the lactose-intolerant person. However, by introducing very small amounts of a high-quality acidophilus product into the system on a daily basis over an extended period of time, the natural production of lactase will be stimulated and the body will begin to take care of this function on its own. Therefore, the optimum way to conquer milk-based allergies is to introduce Megadophilus-Superdophilus, the most potent and viable milk-based L. acidophilus on the market, into the system in small increments (1/16 - 1/8 tsp. once daily) and gradually increase these amounts weekly to the minimum recommended amount of 1/2 tsp. daily.

There is more to the makeup of the healthy microflora than lactobacillus acidophilus. We have already mentioned Bifidobacteria, which is predominantly found in the gastro-intestinal systems of breast-fed infants. Around the age of seven years, the microflora changes from a majority of Bifidobacteria to Lactobacillus acidophilus, which then becomes the predominant strain in the gastrointestinal tract. In approximately 5% of the population, this change never takes place, and we find that these particular people get more positive results from supplementation of Bifidobacteria (Life Start/Bifido Factor).

Actually, I have found that almost every Candida patient can benefit in the beginning by using Bifido Factor/Life Start; in so doing, they repopulate the gastrointestinal tract with the original form of friendly bacteria and, thus, improve the strength of their immune systems. This process can be compared to the difference between building a house on the most solid platform available and building that same house on no platform at all - clearly, the house will last a lot longer on the solidly reinforced platform. The same theory holds true in the case of building your immune system and fighting Candida infections - start with the highest quality supplements available and your results will be that much more positive and long lasting!

It would be highly beneficial for anyone who is just beginning their supplementation program to begin by using both the acidophilus and the Bifidobacteria in order to obtain the maximum benefits. Depending on the type of diet that the person is accustomed to, the ratios of acidophilus to Bifidobacteria are as follows:

- Group #1 - Lacto-vegetarians, Asians, and non-Western cultures: 80% Bifidobacteria and 20% L. acidophilus.
- Group #2 - Individuals on standard Western diet: 80% L. acidophilus and 20% Bifidobacteria.

PRODUCTS ON THE MARKET

There are many different types of supplements currently on the market, all of which make many claims about the superiority of their product over all of the others. Clearly, the consumer must be very discriminating in the choices they make when trying to purchase the most effective products available.

PRODUCT CATEGORIES

To help the consumer focus on the best possible products for them, we have divided the types of acidophilus and Bifidobacteria products that are available into the following categories:

Capsules/Tablets: Again, there is a general lack of potency and stability in these products, although most of the manufacturers of these particular products boost "mega potency" and high stability. The major problem with capsules and tablets is that once they are consumed, the outer shell or capsule triggers the digestive juices to rush to the stomach area, and this means that very few, if any, live microorganisms ever reach the colon, which is where they are supposed to implant. And again, these forms of supplementation are very cost-intensive due to the amounts which need to be consumed. At the usual doses recommended, a bottle of 60 capsules or tablets only lasts 7 days!

Hypo-allergenic/Milk-free/Vegetable-based: As we mentioned earlier, there are clearly many disadvantages to choosing these types of supplements. The processing of these brands of L. acidophilus does great damage to the microorganisms by taking them out of their natural environment, thus eliminating the natural antibiotic properties, and by attempting to artificially boost the potency by suing a process called "centrifuge" or "spinning" the microorganisms. This causes the natural chain to break into many parts, which the manufacturer can then count as separate bacteria when, in actuality, they are simply broken parts of these bacteria. This process injures the microorganisms and severely shortens their natural life span. These products, in particular, are virtually useless to the consumer with severe Candida problems or digestive disorders and should be avoided.

High-potency Powders: Currently, several manufacturers have got their own versions of high-potency L. acidophilus powders on the market, and a few have got compatible high-potency bifido-bacteria products also on the market. In my opinion, these are the most effective forms of supplementation available. And, among these supplements, one particular brand stands out as being the best that money can buy. The manufacturer of these products is the Natren Company, and I will elaborate about these products below.

The Natren Company currently manufactures the most superior and effective L. acidophilus and Bifidobacteria products available, in my opinion. These products are MEGADOPHILUS-/SUPERDOPHILUS, the most efficacious L. acidophilus available, and LIFE START TWO/BIFIDO FACTOR, which is their Bifidobacteria supplement. Both of these products are easily the best around. The L. acidophilus is a highly viable single strain (DDS 1) which produces an extremely effective natural antibiotic, "acidophilin," which was mentioned earlier in the chapter. MEGADOPHILUS/SUPERDOPHILUS is known to inhibit 27 types of bacteria, 11 of which are known pathogens (disease-causing bacteria). It has been shown in research to be very helpful for many skin disorders which stem from digestive problems. It reduces cholesterol levels in the blood, it produces enzymes which increase the effectiveness of the digestive process and produces vitamins in the body which are especially helpful when under stress. In addition, it normalizes the pH within the gastrointestinal system and virtually eliminates excess stomach acid and indigestion discomfort. And, as stated earlier, most people who suffer from lactose intolerance can eliminate this problem by taking daily supplementation of MEGADOPHILUS-/SUPERDOPHILUS. One of the major benefits from MEGADOPHI-LUS/SUPERDOPHILUS supplementation is that continued use can help eliminate Candida albicans (yeast infection) problems. Natren also came out with their own, specially designed applicators which are used when local application of their products are recommended, either vaginally or rectally. Natren's Bifidobacteria bifidum supplement, LIFE START TWO/BIFIDO FACTOR, has been found to be very effective in liver detoxification and, as stated earlier, in helping to cure Candida albicans. This is extremely important, when the fact that the first organ to be attacked by the Candida microorganisms is the liver, is taken into consideration. Regular use of LIFE START TWO/BIFIDO FACTOR also detoxifies the blood by decreasing levels of blood ammonia, free serum phenol, and free amino nitrogen. In addition, benefits are increased nutrient absorption.

Bifidobacteria infantis, the bacteria in Natren's LIFE START, is the first line of immune-system defense for infants and young children. It creates an unfavorable environment for viral and bacterial infections. When taken by pregnant and lactating women, LIFE START will effectively increase the amount of friendly bacteria that is found in breast-milk, which are very often diminished by air pollutants, the chemicals found in our water, food additives, alcohol, and antibiotic treatments. By supplementing the daily diet with a potent, stable product such as Natren's LIFE START, pregnant and lactating women can be assured that they are providing their children with the most pure and effective form of Bifidobacteria available.

All of Natren's products are cultured on pure, high quality milk solids. No hormones, MSG, or other growth enhancers are ever used by Natren to stimulate growth. No artificial methods of boosting potency (such as the centrifuging method used by other companies) are ever used. Natren carefully packs their products in amber colored glass jars, which keeps light and moisture from damaging their products. Natren guarantees the efficacy of every jar of their fine products when used and maintained according to their instructions.

Another important lactobacillus product is the Lactobacillus liquid of GRL. So far it is the best available in fluid on the market. It contains billions of the most viable Lactobacilli. Normal dosis, 1 tbs. after meals. This product is also excellent for vaginal yeast infections-- douche with 1 tbs. Lactobacillus in 3 ounces of water for several evenings.

F. BOOST THE IMMUNE SYSTEM

Just twenty years ago, the question of strengthening the immune system was not an issue. Now the answer to this problem seems to be the best sought secret on our planet.

What insults have we done to our immune system that allow such diseases as AIDS, Leukemia, Herpes Simplex, Systemic Candidiasis (candida yeast overgrowth), recurrent EBV (Ebstein Barr), and CMV (cytomegaly virus) to take their toll on our population? These immune suppressed diseases are reaching epidemic proportions and Systemic Candidiasis has to be put at the top of the list. What are we doing for these diseases now? Our usual approach: we try to take medications to kill the viruses or yeast; we try to find out the way of contamination and, thus, control the spreading; and if one finds a nutritionally-oriented doctor, the patient might be put on an appropriate diet. Unfortunately, the anti-viral medications are not only deficit, they all have very dramatic side effects. Why are we repeating our errors and trying to cure the disease when it is already prevalent? Certainly, the most logical method of combatting a disease is to PREVENT it in the first place.

Every minute of every day wars rage within our bodies. The combatants are so small that we do not even notice these incessant battles. We have evolved legions of defenders, specialized cells that silently rout the unseen enemy. Sometimes the penetration of our defenses by these invaders is successful as is seen in allergic reactions, colds, flu, yeast infections, or to the extreme, AIDS. But, thousands of attempts are repelled thanks to the invisible vigilantes of our immune system.

The human immune system is functioning as a kind of biological democracy, wherein each member has a certain task. These defender white blood cells fall into three groups: the phagocytes, or "cell eaters," and two kinds of lymphocytes, the T and B cells. They only have one objective: identify and destroy all cells that are not part of the human body.

How does the battle begin? As viruses invade the body, some are consumed by the Macrophages (cell eaters). Being the frontline defender, these cells summon Helper T cells to the scene. The Helper T cells are the generals of the troops, identifying the enemy and beginning to multiply. The Helper T cells recruit and activate the Killer T cells who are specialized in killing cells that are invaded by foreign organisms. A second class of defenders called to the war scene are the B cells, residing in the spleen and lymph nodes. The Helper T cells activate the multiplication of these B cells which start forming antibodies.

Meanwhile, some of the viruses are successful enough to invade human cells. Killer T cells will simply sacrifice these cells by chemically puncturing their membranes or walls. The viruses released from those cells will be neutralized by the antibodies, produced by the B cells, which will bind directly to the viral surfaces.

Once the infection is contained, Suppressor T cells halt the activities of the B and T cells, preventing them from going out of control. As a new barrier of defense, Memory T and B cells are left in our blood stream, ready to move when the same viruses would invade our body again.

Of course, the enemy is sometimes very deceptive. Many viruses have found devious methods to escape early detection. Common cold viruses for example, constantly mutate, changing their finger prints. Other viruses are hiding out in healthy cells or what is even worse, are able to kill Helper T cells, the commander in chief of our immune system, therefore short-circuiting this whole defense mechanism.

Aging is also the result of the long term breakdown of the immune system which leads us to the seductive theory that boosting our immune system might also lead to tremendous increases in our lifespan, an overall well-being.

Tremendous improvements have been made in our therapeutic approach for cancer patients. However, unfortunately, cortisone and chemotherapy are also known to suppress the various white blood cells and the immune system, in general. Radiation therapy used on various cancer forms has induced the same detrimental side effect.

It is frightening to see the increasing number of people who are becoming sick from their environment. Pesticides, sprays, leaded gasoline, atomic bomb tests, to mention just a few, have created a vast change in the atmosphere and an increasing number of the population are becoming alarmed.

A third group of offenders are our food ingredients. The amount of preservatives (over 2,700 approved by the FDA) present in our food is outrageous, not to mention the junk food that is being consumed. "Fast food" is common terminology which not only indicates a type of restaurant, but also a lifestyle. We surely do live fast, but we obviously will not live too long this way.

Another group of noxious stimuli to our immune system is almost completely forgotten or largely neglected by our medical society: our emotions. Some people think that emotions cannot have that sort of impact on their bodies and denial is such an easily available defense mechanism.

Before I tell you how to deal with a deficient immune system, I would like to expand a little more about our food.

The authority of the FDA over food additives is derived from the FOOD, DRUG AND COSMETIC ACT OF 1938. Under this Act, the federal government had to prove a substance unsafe before it could prohibit its use in a food. This was changed in 1958 by the FOOD ADDITIVE AMENDMENTS, which states now that a manufacturer must show "proof of a reasonable certainty that no harm will result from the proposed use of an additive." So, now the burden of proving safety has moved from the government to the manufacturer.

By the time this law had passed, a lot of additives were already in use and common additives such as salt, sugar, and spices used for centuries were not even questioned. So we were stuck with a whole group of additives for common use!

And, once they are on the safe list of the FDA, in order then for a chemical to be taken off this list, the FDA must demonstrate the harmfulness of that product.

We have to realize that many additives are purely cosmetic, unnecessary and redundantly used even when substitutes are available. It is not possible here for me to cite the alleged toxicity of thousands of additives that have not been checked for their possibilities of causing birth defects, cancer or other diseases. The oldest one is salt and we know already that over-consumption causes hypertension and heart diseases.

MSG (Monosodium Glutamate) is a flavor enhancer used in numerous products such as processed foods, TV dinners, meats, canned foods, seafood, poultry and crackers. Banned from baby foods, MSG has been found to cause brain damage in lab animals! It is widely used in restaurants and especially in those serving Chinese food. This flavor enhancer modifies food flavor but does not add any flavor on its own.

Today, food colors are used in almost all processed foods. There are about 30 colors that have been approved, half of which are synthetic. Citrus Red #2 and Yellow Dye #5 are two of the more popular ones, found in beverages, ice cream, cereals, oranges and snacks. What to do about these colors? Avoid processed foods containing additives and go back to a more natural diet. Don't be hazardous to your health, eat more natural foods!

So how do we boost the immune system?
1. Start by avoiding, as much as possible, noxious factors such as chemicalized foods, bleached flour, excessive smoking and drinking, chemotherapy and radiation. And, when you are subjected to the above agents, which tells you indirectly that you have not been the greatest supporter for your immune system, you had better try to turn the tables with the following measures.

2. Supplements:

a. ZINC: The thymus shrinks in size and function rather early in life. This will, of course, limit its ability to produce the T-cells. By supplementing with zinc, 50 mg. per day (Zinc Orotate, one tablet a day, GRL), the thymus is effectively bolstered even when begun late in life. Do not forget that zinc is commonly deficient in American diets, particularly among the elderly who need it most. Since it is not uncommon for zinc tablets to cause stomach upset, they are best taken shortly after a meal. Natural sources of zinc are round steak, lamb chops, pork, pumpkin seeds, eggs and mustard. Also, soybeans, turkey, most nuts, peas and berries. There are numerous qualities of zinc supplements on the market. My favorite one is Zinc Orotate, which provides 55 mgs. of elemental zinc. Zinc Orotate seems to be exceptionally well-tolerated and absorbed and is a natural product. Zinc is best tolerated on a full stomach but better absorbed on an empty one. So it is a choice between tolerance of the gastrointestinal system versus absorbability. The supplement is especially indicated in young people suffering from recurrent colds, growth disturbances, flu and allergies, pregnant and lactating mothers and elderly people with prostate risk. The synergism between insulin and zinc is well known. Zinc is the most important mineral for either hypoglycemia or diabetes. Other conditions that improved under zinc supplementation are acne (together with Vitamin A), prostatitis, chronic hair loss, but also anxiety and depression. And, last but not least, sufficient amounts of zinc will ensure recovery from accidents, burns and surgery in record time.

b. IRON: Iron is another mineral with positive effects on the production of T-cells through its involvement with several bacteria killing enzymes. Systemic Candidiasis and Herpes Simplex infections are both conditions which are more prevalent with individuals who are iron-deficient. Take Hemolin tablets, one daily after a meal, which provides 20 mg. Ferrous Sulfate (GRL). Natural sources of iron are pork liver, beef kidney, raw clams, red meat, egg yolks, oysters, nuts, beans, asparagus and molasses.

c.   BETA CAROTENE (GRL): The precursor of Vitamin A, Beta Carotene, is recommended by the American Cancer Society. The advantage of taking this material over Vitamin A is that there is no danger of overdosing since Beta Carotene is converted to Vitamin A only as needed. One capsule, 25,000 I.U., daily is a sufficient dose. Also, remember the list of Beta Carotene foods: mangoes, cabbage, spinach, carrots, greens and sweet potatoes.

d.✱ SELENIUM: Selenium is yet another essential mineral which is associated with cancer prevention and a strengthened immune system. It is known to activate production of co-enzyme Q, which, in turn, stimulates the immune system. Deficiency of selenium causes a reduction of lymphocytes and phagocytes, the latter cells which consume foreign pathogens. A daily dose of 100 mcg. is advised and can be obtained by taking one Algasel tablet daily (GRL). Natural sources are bran, tuna, onions, tomatoes and broccoli.

e.   VITAMIN C: A minimum daily allowance of 4000 mg. Vitamin C is recommended, and if tolerated (absence of diarrhea), up to 20,000 mg. will boost the immune system. Natural sources are citrus fruits, berries, tomatoes, cauliflower, potatoes and sweet potatoes. The best available form are the C crystals of GRL: 1 tsp. provides 3000 mgs. of Vitamin C.

f.   GLOBULINS INJECTIONS: A weekly injection of 3CC gamma globulins is extremely helpful in the beginning.

g. ✳ VITAMIN E: One vitamin stands out as essential in
defending against environmental chemicals, and that
is Vitamin E. For starters, among the anti-oxidants,
it is the most powerful. In other words, it has the
strongest ability to protect against the damage of
chemicals on the cell membrane. It is one of the
most important factors in controlling blood pressure
and protects against heart disease. This precious
nutrient, already scarce in the average American
diet, is easily destroyed by the estrogens in birth
control pills. This leaves the pill-user with even
less Vitamin E required to maintain good health.

Vitamin E is also believed to protect against
certain forms of cancer, especially skin cancer.
Since a woman taking the pill has little or no
protection against cancer-causing molecules in the
air and the UV rays of the sun, she has a slightly
greater risk of developing skin cancer.

If that same patient is smoking and overweight,
the danger of developing a blood clot is alarmingly
high! Vitamin E is an anticoagulant, important in
preventing coagulation of the blood. The addition in
the diet of these patients is absolutely necessary.

It is difficult to obtain Vitamin E in food but
you can find some in cold-pressed cotton seeds,
spinach and eggs.

In an era where hundreds of new chemicals invade
your environment yearly and on the other hand
government agencies are contemplating lowering the
already ridiculously low RDA's, you can be content in
the knowledge that there is a wealth of scientific
evidence in favor of using higher than RDA levels of
Vitamin E. Take 400 I.U. as a daily dosis.

The synergistic action between Vitamin E and
Selenium is well known. Taking both these pills

gives each of these products characteristics they otherwise do not have.

There is one thing to keep in mind concerning your supplements. Do not think that you can find <u>one</u> tablet which contains all of the above. For the potency and dosage necessary, it would be impossible to swallow one tablet which contains the levels mentioned.

3. Acupuncture:

We have two ways of increasing the strength of our immune system. First of all, through acupuncture we can increase the amount of defense energy in our body by stimulating certain points on the body. People with recurrent colds, viral infections, and yeast infections are helped by increasing that kind of energy. The other way is the most important since it involves the stimulation of the spleen organ. This organ, besides its important role in the digestive function, also has a key role in the production of white blood cells, thereby, the key role in our immune system. Through stimulation of spleen points, located on the meridians (pathways), the energy in the spleen organ increases and strengthens our immune system. A well-balanced person will not get sick! One of the theories in Acupuncture, well accepted now, is that stimulating acupuncture points will release endorphins and enkephalins. Both substances are natural pain killers. They also seem to reduce anxiety and create a sense of well-being. Even more startling, some studies suggest that they affect macrophages and T cells, therefore enhancing the immune system. As you see, this ancient art of healing is more important now than ever!

4. Diet:

Cold food and raw food will harm the spleen. The Candida diet is a good example of an immune boosting diet, although in absence of Systemic Candidiasis there is more variety allowed. Steamed vegetables, eggs, fish, chicken, turkey, sweet potatoes and white potatoes, tropical fruits, bread (rye or wheat), soy sprouts, miso, lean meats, with a minimum consumption of beef, buckwheat, millet and oats are all substances of an immune boosting diet. Avoid cold and raw foods since they will transform to "Heat-Damp" in the spleen, decreasing the energy in that organ.

5. Emotions:

Each organ is linked to certain emotions. The spleen (or our immune system) is related to worry and obsession. People with spleen deficiency are typical "Personality Type A": analytical, intelligent, meticulous and fixed in the Freudian anal stage (extreme cleanliness, obsessive, compulsive personality). If you want to minimize insults to the immune system, you had better change this lifestyle!

6. Exercise:

"Mens Sana in Corpore Sano" (a healthy spirit in a healthy body) should be your life slogan. Exercise will move the energy in the meridians, therefore, bringing one into better balance. Exercise may also result in increased levels of INTERLEUKIN-1 and INTERFERON, both of which strengthen our defenses. When helper T cells encounter an enemy, they release a spurt of Interleukin that commands other lymphocytes to multiply.

Following the aforementioned rules, can we be sure to beat the odds in our favor? Of course, none of the above guarantees that we personally will have increased lifespan, just as we have no guarantees that we will not get lung cancer if we do not smoke. However, there is ample evidence that we can bend the odds greatly in our favor with these simple measures. The choice is yours!

It is extremely important to strengthen the immune system while you are eradicating the Candida, otherwise, recurrences of the yeast infection are common and certain! The patient will forever have to follow the diet and use the anti-fungal medications.

G. REPLACE THE MISSING SUPPLEMENTS

A high frequency with a specific constellation of nutritional deficiencies accompanies all forms of chronic Candidiasis. A triad of:

- Magnesium
- Essential Fatty Acid
- Vitamin B6

deficiency appears to be the rule, especially when its toxic or allergic manifestations are present.

1. Abnormal metabolism of Fatty Acids (EFA)

Only a few years ago, the role of Essential Fatty Acids, such as gamma linolenic acid (GLA), was largely ignored by researchers, medical practitioners and nutritionists. With the advent of the prostaglandins (PGs) and the discovery related to their importance to good health, all that has changed. The key ingredient in Evening Primrose Oil, GLA, is effective in treating a diversity of ailments, including acne, arthritis, PMS, overweight conditions, hypertension and a host of other health problems.

Perhaps even more important, primrose oil appears to be one of the most potent agents of preventive medicine of all time. Where does the plant originate from? As it is almost always, it is a rediscovery since the Indians in North America have used it therapeutically for the last five hundred years. Throughout most of its history, the whole plant was used as an herb. It was in 1919 in Germany, that two chemists reported the presence of unusual fatty acids which they named GLA. It was not until the sixties that scientists discovered the high biological potency of the oil. In 1982 the Nobel Prize in Physiology and Medicine was awarded to three researchers instrumental in the discovery of the PROSTAGLANDINS (PGs), whose importance to good health is difficult to overstate. These essential fatty acids are the precursor of the PGs. They are called essential because they cannot be made by the body, and are called "Linoleic Acid" and "Linolenic Acid." They are required for proper membrane structure and function of all body cells.

The body uses linoleic acid to produce GLA, providing things are functioning properly. Unfortunately, a number of facts can prevent this reaction from happening. Among the culprits are: sugar, cholesterol, saturated fats, consumption of alcohol, diabetes, aging and viral infections. Even our deficiencies in our American diet, such as Zinc, Magnesium and C, slow the reaction.

Fortunately, by supplementing the diet with the GLA in Evening Primrose Oil, harmful affects can be eliminated. The oil is NOT a drug. It is a nutritional supplement needed in everybody's diet. A dosis of 40 mgs. GLA, four to six times a day will be of excellent help in combatting most of the above mentioned health conditions.

2. Magnesium

Magnesium still does not get the attention that other minerals receive. However, it is vitally important to our body as it performs many services. There has been enough evidence that sudden heart failures among young men are possibly due to a lack of this mineral. A balance of magnesium and calcium provides a smooth-beating heart.

The magnesium is necessary for proper functioning of the muscles. It works together with calcium (we need twice as much calcium as we do magnesium), but in high doses these two minerals can antagonize each other.

Deficiency of magnesium gives a whole web of symptoms: irritability, anxiety, depression, muscle tremor, muscle twitches and convulsions. Where does this deficiency come from? Intake of diuretics are a major cause! Several of them tend to produce marked levels of magnesium (Hydrochloro-thiazide). Excessive alcohol consumption is another reason. The diet of elderly people is often poor in magnesium and, of course, they are the ones that most commonly take these diuretics.

Often when I mention a deficiency of magnesium to my

patients, they show me previous lab tests that indicate normal serum levels. But magnesium is primarily an INTER-CELLULAR cation, therefore, using serum magnesium levels as a guideline is wholly inaccurate. We need to study the intracellular magnesium, measuring the red-cell magnesium level. However, it is subject to technical difficulties. The Mg load test has been advanced as the most sensitive test of Mg nutriture in patients. The Mg load test is a measurement of the Mg in urine (24 hrs.) after injecting 2cc of Mg.

It is of importance to know that decreased levels of Mg go together with decreased levels of Potassium. Patients with kidney disease, diabetes, colitis ulcerosa, malabsorption and Candida, all require a higher intake of this mineral. These patients would benefit on an intake of 400 to 600 mg. of Mg. Take, by preference, a product where the Mg and Calcium are balanced in one product. ("Kalmaca," GRL)

3.   Vitamin B6

This important vitamin helps assimilate proteins and fats. It prevents various nerve and skin disorders and works as a natural diuretic and muscle pain reliever. Natural sources for the Candida patient are: liver, kidney, heart, cabbage, eggs and beef. 50 mg. daily is a sufficient dosage.

4.   Other nutrient deficiencies

The most common deficiency is the low store of iron, as measured by serum ferritin levels. Iron deficiency is a known predisposing factor to Candida infection, so these low levels should be taken seriously.

Other noted deficiencies are Folate deficiency, Vitamin A (with normal serum carotene), Vitamin C, B12, and Biotin deficiency. Correction of these low levels will reduce the growth of yeast cells.

Another important factor is the synergism or teamwork between proteins and Vitamin A. The body cannot utilize protein without accompanying Vitamin A. Without sufficient amounts of Vitamin A, protein cannot be stored in the major depot, the liver. This vitamin seems to be essential to changing the protein we eat into the protein of which we are made.

Calcium intake will be another necessity, especially for women in the menopause. With the abstinence of dairy products, the intake of calcium is minimal. But there is another reason: high protein diets, such as the Candida diet, may disrupt your calcium balance. Augment your protein intake to 150 grams and you will lose considerable precious calcium in your urine. It is a good idea to increase your intake of calcium and phosphorus substantially while you are on a prolonged protein binge. Take 1500 mg. calcium (2 tablets of 750 mg.) at night.

HOW DO WE KNOW WE ARE BETTER OR HOW DO WE MEASURE THE IMPROVEMENTS?

Does this question surprise you? Not me. Too often I have heard it in practice. It is proper to human nature to forget bad times and to feel only the present. Often, I have to recall to the patients what the original symptoms were, because they tend to focus on the actual problems, sometimes magnifying them. Of course, with the occurrence of new "healing" symptoms, the patient can get confused. Are these healing, die-off or Candida symptoms is another frequently heard question.

There are several methods to measure improvement. The easiest one is to look at all the symptoms involved. It is advised in the beginning to answer a questionnaire similar to the one enclosed in this book (page 137). Even after one month, patients are already surprised when they repeat the questionnaire and see that many of the symptoms have either disappeared or lessened in degree. There is otherwise no way for the patient to remember how s/he felt about a particular disturbance in the body.

A more objective proof is to repeat the blood test if there was one done in the beginning. It is one of the advantages to perform one, because an improved lab test is often the encouragement a patient needs to continue in the right direction. I like the Candida antibody test which will give me three different antibody measurements: IgM, IgA and IgG. Especially the IgM and IgA have to be followed: the IgA, being the "tissue" antibody and the IgM, "the circulating" antibody will decrease with successful therapy, indicating that the Candida cells are leaving organs and blood stream.

Another objective sign, but less expensive is the tongue picture. Looking at the tongue was always a meaningful diagnostic test for our older colleagues, but fell in disgrace with all the modern lab tests available. However, you can hardly find a more objective sign of your health.

For an acupuncturist, it is one of the most important diagnostical steps. What is a normal tongue picture and what do we see with the Candida patient?

Ideally, tongue picture diagnosis should be performed in bright sunlight, in order to avoid false interpretations. Tongue diagnosis gives important and objective information, and gross changes can be distinguished rather easily. A normal tongue, found in a healthy individual, is neither engorged (fat) nor constricted (thin). It has a moderately red color, is relatively wet and has NO COATING ("fur") or a thin, white coating. The tongue is divided into areas which correspond to the different organs. The area important for the yeast patient is the middle part of the tongue. View the tongue in the morning before eating! The tongue picture will constantly change during the day, under the influence of food intake.

The tongue shows different signs with the Candida patient. We see in the middle area of the tongue a white, sometimes yellow coating. The thicker the coating and the more yellow the color, the graver the disease. A favorable prognosis is the yellow color changing into white while the coating is thinning. The tongue in yeast conditions is usually thick. It is not unusual that all the mouth mucosae are covered with the typical white color (trush).

As we can see, there are some ways of recognizing progress although most patients do not need any of the above methods. After one month, 7-step therapy, life is brighter than ever!

7

Psychological Profile

Feelings of frustration, being misunderstood and rejected seem to be part of our life experience. To a Candida patient, these feelings are often magnified; life seldom seems to treat the Candida patient fairly.

In the early childhood experience of the Candida patient, abuse often has been present. The experience of sexual, emotional, or physical abuse are indications of a traumatic childhood, in which emotional nourishment, encouragement in goal-setting, or simply the coherence of a healthily functioning family are absent.

This fear inducing environment influences one's immune system in a weakening manner, leaving one susceptible for invasion of diseases. Ancient medicine practices, such as Acupuncture and Homeopathy, have indicated the relationship between physical illnesses and emotions. According to the philosophy of Acupuncture, each emotion is linked to a certain organ. Fear, for instance, will decrease the energy in the Kidney organ, worry and pensiveness will do the same in the Spleen. A sudden, extreme shift in one's emotions, thus, will effect one's equilibrium, leaving one temporarily open to the invasion of viruses, bacteria, yeast cells, or in the worst case, to the onset of debilitating disease. A good example is the occurrence of rheumatoid arthritis after a sudden, extreme fearful event: a divorce, sudden death in the family, loss of a job are all situations related to extreme anxiety and fear. This negative emotion will deplete the energy in the Kidney organ, and usually leads to the onset of the first arthritis attack a couple of months later. What makes it even worse, deficiency of energy in the Kidney organ leads to more fear and anxiety, pulling the patient in a vicious circle.

What fear does to the Kidney, worry does to the Spleen. People get obsessed with the past, isolate themselves, leading to a crash down of energy in the Spleen.

What follows next is the common nightmare of the Candida patient. As a child, most of these patients are subjected to an increased antibiotic intake and our modern diet with preservatives and sugars. Most of the symptoms will appear a couple of years later, but sometimes immediate yeast-related signs surface: mood swings, depression or suicidal tendencies. The sudden mood swings are the most startling symptoms. Patients look and act joyful at 10 a.m. and are threatening to kill themselves by 2 p.m. We can understand the skepticism and disbelief of professionals and family; nobody, not even the patient, expects these sudden variations. At the end, the patient self is convinced that s/he had become crazy: it is the only possible answer on this yo-yo behavior.

You know where the real problem of the Candida patient starts? Most of these victims, especially in the beginning stages, look too healthy, too handsome... In fact, they look too good to have any kind of disease! This is the Catch-22: outwardly, it does not look like a disease. And, for the text-book physician, looking for objective signs, he hardly finds them. How can you see "fogginess" in the brain, burning urination, severe PMS symptoms, decreased attention span... The most, the patient looks depressed. "Go shopping," "Eat a cake," (how ironic) or "Take a short vacation," are frequently heard and well meaned advices.

The emotion though, that predominates this disease, is ANGER! All Candida patients have a reservoir of anger, mostly deeply hidden. There is a need to understand the origin of anger and to seek means of dealing with the factors involved. Do not believe that this anger will always show in violent behavior. There are other levels of manifestation of anger: colitis ulcerosa, hypertension, eczema, migraine attacks, depressions and suicidal tendencies can be expressions of this emotion. Most patients will not even admit that they are angry. However, a lot of their expressions imply underlying anger. "I am bitter the way my doctor treats me" or "I am fed up the way my husband denies this problem," "It irritates me, I cannot get any explanation from anyone" are only anger in disguise. In fact, anger, frustration and irritability are all emotions linked in acupuncture to an imbalance in the Liver organ.

However, I feel that it makes more sense to recognize and accept the anger as such. Patients who find no place to put their anger, are ridden by guilt, which offers no relief. Letting the anger out, little by little, is like relieving some steam. Somebody in a support group said, "Since nobody seems to understand my problem, I stopped talking about it." She might not be aware of it, but there is an immense amount of anger behind this passive behavior.

Another manifestation of hidden anger in almost every Candida patient is bodily reactions to it. An almost constant symptom in these patients is the pain in the neck and shoulder region. We know the expression, "You are a pain in the neck," these patients actually have pain in the neck because they ARE angry and they refuse to accept it or are not allowed to bring the anger outwardly.

Of course, this chronic disease solicits anger as well from the patient as from the rest of the family, especially the partner. The patient may build up the anger for all kinds of reasons. They feel constantly rejected, are always questioned and doubted about the existence of this disease, and simply because they are outside the mainstream and do not get their share of the world's excitement and rewards. The partner resents this disease immensely because it makes him a prisoner in his own house, without having the disease. They are inconvenienced by their partner's illness, leading to feelings of frustration and resentment.

Why do some of these patients turn out well, while others go completely on the wrong track, socially and healthwise? I believe that we use the frustrations of growing up to form a certain force that will be constructively for the first group, but destructively for the latter one. Candida patients, as a group belonging to the most abused ones, unfortunately use that energy to manifest their anger, isolating them as "trouble makers," "nuts," and "lazy people." Crying spells in a Candida patient are nothing else but an expression of their anger, it is, in fact, in a lot of cases, their sole outlet for it. At least it might trigger more sympathy than overt hostility and irritability, but in essence, it will be the same. During their whole lives, anger has been built up, there is a whole storage that needs only a small stimulus to erupt in a volcano of stored-up emotions, unfortunately, easily put on the wrong persons. Children have an easier time expressing their anger, directly towards the person involved. My son, at the ripe age of six, expresses his anger towards me very easily, "I hate you." It does not make him a monster, all he is saying is, "I am angry at you."

Returning to the Candida patients, their mood swings can turn into suicidal thoughts. Again, this is the ultimate form of their bottled anger, turned against the self. The anger and frustration can be so big, that they are literally "trying to kill themselves," mainly as an ultimate expression of their anger and dejection, turned inward.

What can the patient do to channel this anger in a positive force? First, the patient has to accept that there is anger. It is my experience that most Candida patients do this. Their first sentence to me is often, "I am angry at all these doctors..." For them to identify the source of this emotion, is not so difficult, at least not a first hand.

Doctors who are not able to diagnose the disease are the main culprits for their "lost years." However, there might be some displacement involvement. I am sure some of these doctors deserve the anger they get for being narrow-minded and incompassionate. It is typically for abused children to feel guilty. "They must have attracted this abuse because of their behavior." However, since this anger had no outlet in childhood, the doctor-patient relationship is perfectly suited to let some steam off and to direct some anger at another person.

Of course, many Candida patients know exactly why they are angry. They have been wandering around for years, suffering with pain, depression, fatigue, but the man they turned to for help, their doctor, failed to recognize the source of their problems. Once the patient realizes it was NOT "all in his head," and lost, therefore, years of his life, s/he naturally berates all those doctors for not supplying the help they need.

How can we deal with this anger?

We might confront those doctors that failed to recognize our condition. However, in case of the Candida patient, it might be a catch-22: still now, most doctors deny the existence of this disease, adding fuel to our anger. So, it might be necessary to find some other outlets for our emotions. Do not fall into the trap that you are angry! Better communication with the direct family to create an immediate support group is a satisfactory solution. And, it is an excellent idea to take the spouse along to Candida support groups, to meet other people with the same problems.

Having gone through these different steps should really solve the problem. Unfortunately, life is a lot more complex, and theory does not always translate into practice. However, dealing better with your anger will avoid from turning this negative feeling against yourself, therefore, hampering your full recovery. Drive, determination and a positive mental attitude will prevent breakdowns.

The real key to resolve most of the problems for any patient is good communication. That's what the next chapter is all about. Mark Fowler and Gloria Axelrod explore useful tips for the Candida patient to overcome most of the painful situations they are confronted with.

One more important psychological aspect of this disease: patients that are recovering, or even completely healed, have a hard time to let go of sickness and reach for new responsibilities and vitality. Friends will no longer need to support their weakness, they sometimes get less attention and sympathy. They may also lose some of their celebrity status, since "Candidiasis is in the news." Some patients try to get by in spite of feeling OK, simply because it is too scary after all these years to face the real competitive, neurotic world. Patients have to take a solid stand to change, to move on with their lives and leave behind this old foe, Candida. I must say though, a very positive aspect of these patients is their willingness to help other people with the same condition. I have never seen a group more eager to help fellow sufferers overcome the different difficult barriers in their recovery. I guess this disease changes you forever!

8
Coping Confidently With Candida

FRUSTRATIONS OF AN ILLNESS

After several mornings of waking up tired, grumpy and apathetic, you decide that nothing is working out. You're not getting any better. Your allergies are acting up, you're not concentrating properly, you have less and less energy.

When you finally see the doctor, after rushing to get there and then having to wait, you explain your depressing condition. The doctor says there doesn't seem to be any justification for your unusual symptoms. He asks if they might be psychological in nature.

Though he phrases it nicely, it still boils down to "your problems are all in your head." Frustrated and disheartened, you realize this situation is life-threatening to you--but you wonder how you can make that clear to anyone else? It's often hard to get doctors' assistance for a disease they can't see or identify. Much easier to have a broken limb!

Candida is not easily treatable because many of the symptoms are vague. Also, as discussed in the body of this book, the medical profession is only beginning to accept its full scope and impact.

You don't tend to group Candida with life-threatening illnesses like the ominous heart disease, cancer, arthritis or AIDS. But any illness, even a headache, disrupts your life when it invades your own person. People needed to help--doctors, therapists, friends, lovers, family, bosses--want to participate, to come to the rescue. But they don't know how.

Communication is challenging because each person's frame of reference is different--and constantly changing. When you add unique Candida symptoms, the stress of illness, and the generally apathetic medical environment, the Candida person is in an exceptionally difficult position.

GETTING HELP

Assume Responsibility

The question is: How do I get help? The first step is to be responsible--ask for it. As one of Doctor DeSchepper's patients said, "We have a responsibility. We got ourselves sick, we've got to get ourselves well. I had to go through three doctors before I found Luc."

When your health is at stake, you must take charge of guiding others to help you help yourself. A perfect example of the situation we are discussing occurred several years ago to Mark. It was not Candida-related, but it was definitely life-threatening.

Mark was visiting a woman friend for the first time, and was waiting for her to get ready to go out. He was sitting in the kitchen waiting, while her two teenagers were in the living room watching TV. They had only just been introduced. Eating some potato chips, Mark accidentally inhaled a piece of chip.

After several attempts to remove the chip, he realized he could not breathe or speak. Fear was the first reaction: I don't know anyone here, how do I tell them what's going on, how much time do I have?

Realizing he truly needed help, he walked over to the teenage boys. Picking the closest boy, Jack, who seemed also the most friendly, he took Jack's hand, strongly but gently, looked into his eyes very seriously and mouthed silently, "I need your help."

He guided the boy up from the chair, and turned around. Mark then took Jack's hands and arms and put them around his chest.   He motioned Jack to pull his hands hard into Mark's chest...the Heimlich Maneuver.

Jack did it, and it worked the first time!   Mark could breathe again.   He thanked Jack, hugged him, and went on to have a wonderful evening, glad to be alive.

Well, great story, but what may you ask does this have to do with Candida?   Everything.   Mark found that when he took responsibility to ask for someone's help, gently and calmly, he got it.

Asked later why he so easily responded to Mark's request, Jack said he knew Mark was serious and needed help.   Jack felt he had no other choice but to respond.

Become Partners

Jack and Mark became partners--a team.   Those of us with Candidiasis, Mark included, need teamwork and information. Mark had read about the Heimlich Maneuver, but was not trained in it.   You may not be trained in any particular therapy, either, but you have your own symptoms, experiences, readings and discussions to draw on.

The two most important means of support for you as a Candida patient are a successful and satisfying working relationship with your physician, and the reinforcement and understanding of those closest to you: your family and friends.

While we primarily address physician and family giving you some techniques that will help, these same techniques can be used with waiters, waitresses, bosses and medical insurance personnel, as they are basically universal.

Probably one of the hardest things for all of us to do is receive help.   "I can handle it, I don't need help," seems to be a big part of our personal philosophy.   We are quick to help others, but slow to ask for it ourselves.

The key is: We are usually ready to help the other guy. Let's take advantage of that situation and give them the change to be happy--by helping us.   But, first we must make it clear we NEED help.

Let's take a situation common to all Candida patients who may have tried several therapies and 'cures' but still have the same symptoms and who don't seem to be getting well.

WORKING WITH YOUR PHYSICIAN

When the initial treatment doesn't work, our first reaction might be to strike out at the doctor for not 'curing' us. It is here that a little preparation comes in handy.

Be Prepared

1. MAKE A LIST of exactly what you did since you last met the doctor. Did you follow your diet, prescription, etc.? Did you notice any unusual symptoms or habit changes? Try to crystallize what happened so that you can give that information to the doctor. He is not a mind reader, and the only way he can help is to get all the information.

After you have made your lists, read them over to see if there is anything additional that might help. Next, outline what you want to talk to the doctor about, for example: goals, concerns, questions, or problems.

This may seem like a lot of work, but being prepared is critical to giving and receiving meaningful information. It also helps to relieve your anxiety and concern because these thoughts, questions, ideas, feelings are no longer swimming around in your head--they're down on paper!

Armed with your list, you can meet your doctor with added confidence.

2. Explain that you have all this information as soon as you meet with your doctor. (It would be appropriate to mention this when you telephone for your appointment. But messages often get lost or garbled.) Ask if he has the time to discuss it now. He might prefer to reschedule or suggest an alternative. Explain that this is not a routine follow-up, it is a major point in your therapy when you believe change is necessary. It is IMPORTANT to you, and your doctor needs to realize that.

3. State your overall objective and your concern about reaching it. It is important to keep it simple and to the point. The following paragraph might be your introduction:

"Dr. Smith, I seem to be feeling worse, and I'm experiencing some unusual symptoms. I'm very concerned about this, and about my therapy in general. I've made a list of my symptoms, questions and concerns. Do you have the time today to help me with it?"

You have stated your problem, that you're prepared to work together, and you're asking for help. The ball is in the doctor's court as to how s/he can help. You and the doctor can develop options TOGETHER as to how to handle the time scheduling.

Let's review the above suggestions:
1. Be prepared by making a list of concerns and goals.
2. Let the other persons know your objective.
3. Solicit their help, and let them know you're in it together.

Three Sentence Rule

You don't want to bombard the listener with too much information. To help you with this, there is a technique we call "the three sentence rule." It can help you present information simply, clearly and, most importantly--with few words.

When you have so many things to say, it's hard not to say them all at once, especially at such an emotionally challenging time. If you can keep your communications to small digestible bites of information and wait for feedback, you have a better chance for success.

Not simple, you say. You're right--it does take practice. Fortunately, because we think faster than we talk, we have time to do some editing in our heads.

In the FIRST SENTENCE, state the subject you want to discuss. Next, ADD A SENTENCE that will start to clarify that subject. Third, ASK FOR FEEDBACK. You'll begin to get a feel for your listener's interest, and whether there's enough time to explore more deeply.

Take a minute to review the sample conversation with Dr. Smith. As you go through the paragraph, you will notice that sentence one brings up the subject of unusual symptoms. The second sentence stresses that the symptoms and the therapy are a concern. The third sentence expands on the topic and asks the doctor whether there is time to discuss these concerns. It says a great deal in a short period of time.

This technique looks simple, but it takes time to get comfortable with it. Be patient with yourself. Give it time and practice. We have found that our students, just by trying the three sentences, become more clear and concise. By editing their material, they are encouraging their listeners to respond.

To review the Three-sentence Rule:
1. Sentence one - state your subject
2. Sentence two - say something about the subject
3. Sentence three - ask for feedback

Asking Clarifying Questions and Listening for the Answers

After you have presented your situation, wait and listen to what the doctor has to suggest. Your doctor might say, I'll take whatever time is necessary to help now. You are a valued patient and I know this has been a difficult time for you."

On the other hand, s/he might just say "I've come to the conclusion that there's not much I can do. I'm as stumped as you are with your situation. I think I need to recommend another doctor for you." Whatever the response, it is vital that you take responsibility for GETTING MORE INFORMATION.

This means ASKING QUESTIONS, for increasing your information and clarifying your understanding.

By making sure you understand what the doctor has to say, you let him/her know that you are interested in listening. Also, you have increased your chances of the doctor's listening to you. We've all seen two people who have, instead of a conversation, two alternating monologues.

You can change the monologue pattern, however, by giving the doctor a chance to speak--and RISK being the listener! The information is important for you in order to digest instructions on prescriptions, dietary considerations, work habits, amount of sleep. The clearer your understanding, the better your chances for getting well.

Writing things down is essential. It is very difficult to remember a lot of new information, especially if it is technical or emotional. We know one physician who hands his patient a pad and pencil just as he begins to give his instructions. He wants to be sure the patient gets it right. He then reviews it to verify that what you wrote was what he said. Writing things down in the doctor's presence also convinces him you are really listening.

With listening skills, practice and a positive attitude, you can help your physician recognize your life-threatening situation. You begin to take charge of your own recovery.

Key Words

In order to take your notes more effectively and assure yourself that you are getting all the information, there are several additional listening techniques for you to try. The first is KEY WORDS.

Key words are words or phrases that appear to be stressed by the talker, are unusual or unknown to you, or are emotional or technical in nature. Key words need to be verified so that you're sure you understand them. If Dr. Smith says, "Mary, you need to eat smaller meals more often during the day," there are several important key words to address.

The first is NEED. Why do you need to? What is the reason for not eating at regular meal times? The second is SMALLER. Well, how small? The third is MORE. Three more? Six more? It is critical to get ALL the information in order to understand thoroughly.

How do you use key words? ASK the speaker what they mean and how they affect you. "I don't understand. What do you mean by small?," "I'm confused. Why do I need to do this?"

In asking your questions, it is important to take responsibility for your own misunderstanding or confusion. "I don't understand," is easier for the other person to relate to than "YOU are not being clear." Emphasizing working together to get correct information helps you gain the support you so desperately need.

Paraphrasing

The second technique is "PARAPHRASING." Paraphrasing is restating in your own words what you believe the person said.

Saying something your way often helps you to understand it better. PLANNING to paraphrase helps you focus your attention so that you can be on the lookout for key words. It also demonstrates your listening efforts.

An extra benefit is giving the SPEAKER a chance to add or subtract from his or her statement, or to say it more specifically. Not all of us speak in perfectly edited sentences, containing our precise meaning!

With paraphrasing, you and the speaker become partners and team players, and establish a better appreciation of each other and the problem you are trying to solve.

For example, Dr. Smith might say, "We are not sure how severe your Candida is. We'll have to run several more tests over the next two weeks. In the meantime, we want you to go on a special diet that is high in protein and low in carbohydrates. We also suggest that you exercise at least three times a week."

You might respond, "Let me make sure I understand: Your diagnosis shows that I need more tests, a diet and special exercises. Is that correct?" Obviously, there is a great deal of specific information to learn, and the paraphrasing has given you a starting point.

From here, you can use your other skills such "key words," "asking questions," and, of course, more "paraphrasing" in order to find out everything you need to know. Remember, get information. The more information you have, the fewer misunderstandings you will have to contend with. The net result is you get better faster.

Assumptions

A third technique is "checking out your assumptions." Historically, communication experts have told us not to "assume." However, we believe the assuming is not the problem; it is acting on our assumptions as though they were facts that gets us into trouble.

Assuming is a natural process. Where would we be if a scientist never made a hypothesis, which is just a sophisticated assumption?

How can we make assumptions work for us instead of against us? We can use our assumptions as a springboard to open up new and creative options for our current situations and problems, the way scientists examine a new theory. By checking and verifying our ideas, we can use them for a better understanding of the speaker and of ourselves.

"Checking out assumptions" is similar to paraphrasing--we are confirming parts of the speaker's conversation. We want to know what the speaker is really saying. We all have vivid imaginations and varied frames of reference, and can hear strikingly different meanings and possibilities in the same data.

Making assumptions can be great fun. The central ingredient, however, is allowing yourself the luxury to be wrong, silly, creative, maybe even a little off the wall. No great achievement, whether financial, scientific, or political, was successful without controversial ideas, mistakes and false starts. If you remember this, you may not worry about "looking dumb." You will be able to disclose and verify your assumptions--and get valuable information.

We would not have had the opportunity to write this chapter for Luc's book if we had not assumed that communication was important to helping Candida patients and that we might be able to be of assistance.

How do we use assumptions? When Dr. Smith said, "We are not sure how severe your Candida is. We'll have to run several more tests," you can make a number of assumptions. You might feel that Dr. Smith does not understand your case. You might believe that this process is never going to end. You can feel that you have to take time off from work for tests you think you don't need. The list can go on and on.

However, these assumptions are perfect grist for the mill in your ongoing dialogue with your doctor. If you do not clear these up, you run the risk of doing things wrong, doing too much, or undergoing unnecessary procedures.

These assumptions are SIGNALS to you to get more information. They are an opportunity to learn more about yourself and use your new information appropriately. This takes a bit of courage, however.

It takes courage and some diplomacy to let your doctor know if you feel he is not on track with you. You might start by saying, "Dr. Smith, I think I've been a little unclear with you. First of all, I don't remember whether I told you I was already on a high protein, low carbohydrate diet and I'm exercising three times a week. So, I'm assuming I am not communicating properly. Let's see if there are other areas we need to review."

Another response might be, "Dr. Smith, I feel that this therapy is going on forever. I just don't see any end in sight. And I'm not enthusiastic about all this new work," or, "Dr. Smith, I can't see how I am going to be able to do everything you're recommending, and still work full time."

With these ideas or assumptions out in the open, both you and your doctor can begin to develop ALTERNATIVES. Working as a team, you can create a more structured and defined program that is understandable and has an end in sight.

For example, you might devise your diet and exercise program so that you have more time. It could become a family affair instead of your project exclusively. But, it will not get resolved unless it's brought our into the open with everyone cooperating.

The key to checking assumptions is being willing to say what's on your mind. Be sure to do this without accusing the other person of not listening, being unclear or manipulative.

Then, when you get home and begin to act on any new instructions, you won't find yourself saying, "Oops, is this what he really meant?" You'll feel better if you've said that in his office. You'll have his corroboration and support right from the start. You both win. Together you can help each other create a mutually agreeable plan.

To review the Listening Techniques:

1. Identify "key words or phrases" and ask questions to clarify them.

2. Paraphrase or feed back to the speaker in your own words what you feel s/he is saying.

3. Verify your assumptions no matter how unusual they might seem to be to you.

4. Take responsibility for what is going on with you. Let others know so that there is no confusion.

If, after you've tried all our techniques and you're still not getting the support and help that you need, it is time to consider a new physician. However, please do not look at the time and energy you have spent as wasted. You have learned new ways to communicate, you have learned more about yourself and your illness, and you have a clearer understanding of what you need from your doctor.

Armed with this information, you can now embark on finding a physician who can help. You have new skills and you can use them to make the most of your new doctor/patient relationship. Remember, life is a creative process and your Candida is no exception. So take advantage of your information and your skills to get yourself well.

ASSISTANCE FROM FAMILY AND FRIENDS
The major difference between working with family or friends

and your doctor is that the doctor is there to work with you. It is a professional relationship in which you are to receive a service.

Your family and friends are not a service organization. They have their own lives and their own problems. To get their support and assistance requires consideration for their needs as well as yours. The first thing to realize is that it's very difficult for them to understand and appreciate a disease they've never had, can't see, and never even heard of!

Second, if you're having a hard time expressing what you need or how you feel, they are have an equally difficult time understanding you. They want to HELP, but they just may not know how.

Tough Times

With any disease, there are a lot of difficult or tough times. These might include not feeling well enough to go to work, even though you have a special meeting that day. It might be not feeling up to going to a family outing that you, your spouse and children have planned for a long time. You might not be open to having sexual relations because you do not have the energy or your don't feel attractive.

In addition, we often have tough times that do not relate directly to our physical symptoms. These could be situations where we feel we don't have the skills to deal with a particular circumstance. Going to lunch with the boss and having to order a special meal; or, having to tell a neighbor that his chemical spray is giving you a major allergy attack. This is especially true when these situations are completely new to you.

Needless to say, times like these can be frightening and stressful. "What will my boss think of me?" "My neighbor probably thinks I'm crazy," "My spouse will think I'm not in love anymore." All these can be typical reactions, and difficult for everyone involved.

But as the problem comes from within with us, so does the solution. We need everyone's understanding and support, which we can get by listening to them, and helping them listen to us.

Helping People Get Ready to Listen

We often assume that family and friends are available to us whenever we want to talk. Maybe familiarity allows us to take their attention for granted. We believe it is our responsibility to be sure friends and family are READY to help us.

The best and most direct way to find out is to ASK. You might say to your spouse, "I need to talk to you. When do you think we could have 15 to 20 minutes of uninterrupted time?" Or, "My allergies are just killing me. I think part of it is cigarette smoke. Could we have some time to ourselves to talk about it?"

Using the "three sentence rule" (to recap: main point first, clarify briefly, ask for feedback) you have let the other person know what you want to talk about. Make it clear that when they are READY, you would like their assistance. Finding out whether people are ready to talk is a good daily habit, not only for life threatening diseases. When making either a business or social telephone call, it is considerate to ask whether this is a convenient time to talk.

The same consideration holds true in dealing with your Candida. If you need a ride to the doctor, don't wait until the last minute to find out who is available. Please, ask for help in advance! People need the time and the energy to prepare--except, of course, in an emergency.

But an on-going situation, like Candida, is usually not an emergency. You have to manage and plan for it.

Does this sound like just plain common sense? Well, good communication is often just that--consideration and common sense.

To review: HELPING others to be ready to listen to you:

1.   Plan ahead, know what your needs are likely to be.
2.   Let the person(s) know what you need to talk about.
3.   Ask them when they have the time to discuss this and set aside the time.

Getting Help

Having set the stage for your meeting, you can now begin to communicate your situation. Here we go back to our four standbys: "three sentence rule," "key words," "paraphrasing," and "checking assumptions."

Please consider, too, a wonderful aid that Nature has provided: your ability to modulate your voice. Tone of voice, like a smile, can go a long way toward producing a "helping" atmosphere.

In a "tough time" with your neighbor, a good place to start might be: "Harry, I need your help. I think the chemicals you're using on your lawn are affecting me. My allergies are so much worse since you started your weekly spraying. I was wondering if we could work something out together. What do you think?"

In getting help, it is important to remember that there are many possible solutions. Starting our with, "Harry, if you don't stop using those chemicals on your lawn, I'll sue you," may only get you a punch in the nose.

If you want HELP, it really means THEIR help...a plan they have worked on with you.

The next step is to GET INFORMATION. You might find out that Harry has finished the lawn spraying for this year. You might work out something for next spring. You might find out that Harry has been spraying in the afternoon when the wind is up. Maybe he could spray at night. There are many possible solutions. This is your chance to find them together.

Options

Between you, you can discuss possible options and discover

a solution that can work for everybody. Here is where you use "key words," "paraphrasing," and "assumptions." With these tools, we can seek new information that can help solve the problem.

Just to review these listening techniques:

1. Identify "key words or phrases" and ask questions to clarify them.
2. Paraphrase or feed back to the speaker, in your own words, what you feel he or she is saying.
3. Verify your assumptions no matter how unusual they might seem to be to you.
4. Take responsibility for your condition, and let others know about it so that they are less confused.

Working Together

Our students and clients have been amazed to discover that spending some extra time to explore options can produce quick results. A brainstorming session can offer a wealth of information. Here's how it works: You and your partners say whatever idea or plan comes into your heads, no matter how wild, innovative, outlandish it may be. No fair passing judgment--that comes later!

The first reaction many people have to this idea is that it will take too much time. It can--at first. But it saves time by preventing confusion and bad feelings later on. It often helps YOU feel better faster, and everyone else is happy to have played a part in your success.

An important benefit of this process is that it helps the listener appreciate your difficulties. It prevents a lecture or a long-winded dissertation, and becomes an idea they can relate to, within THEIR frame of reference. It is a process to discover something recognizable in THEIR background. It also helps remove the "If I haven't heard of it, it doesn't exist" attitude.

This takes a good deal of patience and understanding. But if you really need the person's help, it's worth it. Find out whether they have ever been so sick, they could not function. Did they ever have something that was so hard to diagnose that no one would believe they were actually ill.

"Jean, if you have a moment, would you be interested in knowing what my problem is?" This may be one way to start the "working together" process.

If they do show an interest, keep your explanation short and simple. You might say, "I got Candida from taking too many antibiotics when I was sick last summer. It upset the natural balance between the bacteria and yeast in my body. Have you ever taken medicine you thought was going to help but actually made you sicker?"

You might find out that when your neighbor was a child, s/he had a very serious illness that the doctors could not resolve. When the family moved to another town, the symptoms went away. The doctors there discovered that chemicals from a factory's smokestack had been causing an irritation.

You might discover that there are many people with undiagnosed ailments--and that some of them are actually Candida. Then you might be the one doing the helping.

Most people are ready, willing and able to lend a hand, especially if they are involved in DEVELOPING the solution.

To review: To Work Together Better:

1. Maintain an atmosphere of HELPING and being willing to receive help.
2. Emphasize "getting more information," ask clarifying questions.
3. Let the listeners in on the difficulties. Try to relate to something they may have experienced.
4. Take advantage and appreciate people's energy generated by their participation in the process of working out a solution...the successful culmination of brainstorming.

The Real World

Candida can turn normal everyday happenings into difficult

problems......problems unique to Candidiasis:

For example: You have been invited to the home of one of your spouse's friends for an elegant dinner party. You would love to go, but you are afraid of not being able to eat much of the food. You don't want to be embarrassed. But it is very important to your spouse for your both to be there.

What are your options? You could get sick the day of the dinner and not be able to go. You could bring your own food. You might eat first so that you nibble during the meal and avoid any yeast producing products.

But these ideas are yours alone. They don't consider your host and hostess. There might be some alternatives you might not have thought about. The only way to find out, however, is to ASK.

One possibility is to call your host or hostess and talk about it. "Mary, I was delighted to receive your invitation to dinner, but I have an eating problem. Do you have a few minutes to talk?" With that, you are on your way. "My doctor has me on a very strict diet. I would love to come but this diet is so limiting. Do you have any thoughts on how we could work this out?"

From there, you can begin to explore options. Your host or hostess might enjoy the challenge of creating a dish especially for you. Or, maybe the whole meal would be geared to the type of food you can eat--something new for everyone! If it is an informal get-together, you might bring along something for yourself that you and your host have worked out. The options are only limited by the interests and imaginations of the people working together.

To review: In order to be most effective in this type of situation:

1. Ask for HELP; let the person know your situation in advance.

2. Keep your communications short and informative, use the "three sentence rule."

3. Maintain an attitude of HELPING.

4. Solicit your listener's ideas and support a team-work environment.

You can use these techniques in other family and friend situations. Most of the time they work, although they can sometimes be difficult to orchestrate. The most important thing is to RISK the difficulties of finding the help you need to get better--and enjoy yourself along the way.

by

G. Axelrod Ed.M.

&

M. Fowler Cmc, Cpa

Conclusion

There is no doubt that we are facing an important stage in our health. Emotions, hereditary factors, medications, food abuse and environmental laxity have left our immune systems weakened. Diseases such as EBV, CMV, Herpes Simplex, Hypoglycemia, Candidiasis, Leukemia and AIDS have so many symptoms in common because they start from the same point on our freeway to destruction: a total suppressed immune system. Many patients suffering from Candidiasis in the early stages of disease will die in hospitals with the diagnosis of Leukemia or AIDS. Candidiasis is a disease to stay here for a long time unless we are willing to make drastic changes in our lifestyle. And, it is no big help that 90% of the medical profession does not recognize the syndrome or brushes the matter under the carpet by claiming it is "a fad." However, I am confident that we will turn the odds because I am confident in the patients. Under their pressure, we, as a medical community, will be forced to look into this issue.

If there is one good aspect about this disease, it is that we will have to change our lifestyles: patients going through the rigorous diet, the self study of their inner being, the heavy emotions they have to go through such as rejection, isolation, depression, anger and frustration, will forever stay on the right track! A disease such as Candidiasis stays with you for the rest of your life. For any Candida patient with the right mind, it will not be too difficult to fight abuse in the food industry and environment. We have no choice: we get the disease or the disease gets us!

Is Candidiasis a deadly disease? Looking at the mechanism of Candidiasis, it is clear that we get the disease because our immune system is suppressed. Once the yeast cells spread to the blood stream and the organs, our immune system reacts by forming antibodies and becomes eventually exhausted. The next step is the contraction of all kinds of viral diseases such as CMV and EBV (Ebstein Bar virus), Herpes Simples I and II. More down the same road, people will contract leukemia, cancer and AIDS.

Studies performed in Europe showed that gastrointestinal x-rays performed within 4 weeks of death were normal in 11 of 14 patients in spite of the presence of severe Candida esophagitis at autopsy. None of those patients were endo-scoped because the diagnosis of Gastrointestinal Candida was never considered.

The antemortem diagnosis of Candida has been very diffi-cult in the past. Mostly, the diagnosis was never considered or these patients were frequently ill due to the complica-tions of the medications. The fact that nutrition is practically ignored at medical schools did not help.

Candida is frequently found in the gastrointestinal tract of normal people. Especially elderly people seem to harbor more fungi and less lactobacilli. Using stool cultures, we have to keep in mind that the pathogen phase of gastro-intestinal candidiasis is associated with the presence of mycelia in the stools.

As already mentioned, the Candida is most frequently present in the esophagus of the patient. Hence, an endoscopy is the best single method, at least for the classical physician, for diagnosing esophageal moniliasis.

The holistic doctor does not have to rely on this rather unpleasant method. Because stool cultures and endoscopies are not performed by the classical textbook doctor, at least in case of CANDIDIASIS, the case is closed as far as the medical community is concerned. I do not know who is included in this "community," but count me out. How can you give fair consideration to a diagnosis and therapy when the case is closed? This is so true, not just with Candida, but with many innovative ideas in the healing arts. I believe that scientists like Linus Pauling win Nobel Prizes because they DO remain open to possibilities that the ordinary researcher has "closed the case on." It is true, you can draw a few blanks that way, but some mighty worthwhile contributions to the betterment of mankind can also come along and just one of them is worth a lot of disappointments and failures.

Of all the professionals that need to remain open to new possibilities and unique techniques and methods, the medical profession tops the list. Let us not scoff at "unproven" nutritional therapies, vitamin programs and alternative forms of medicine. And, let us return to our oath of Hippocrates, the father of medicine: "NON NOCERE", "You will NOT harm."

Appendices

1. A self-scoring questionnaire
2. Health Food Stores & Restaurants
3. Sources of Help
4. Practical Treatment Plan
5. Recipes

APPENDIX 1: DO I SUFFER FROM THIS DISEASE? A SELF SCORING TEST.

It is easy for anyone to fill this questionnaire in, to have a fairly accurate idea if he/she suffers from the Candida Syndrome. If you answer at least 75% 'yes' on the following questions, yeast-connected health problems are almost certainly present.

A. PAST MEDICAL HISTORY

                                                           YES   NO

1. Have you ever been suffering in the past or are you now, from diseases such as:
   - Hypothyroidy?
   - Hypoglycemy?
   - Diabetes mellitus?
   - Cancer in any form?
   - Burns?
   - Ferriprive anemia?

2. Have you ever been subjected to:
   - Operations?
   - Catheterizations?
   - Intake of cytostatic (anti-cancer therapy), radiations?

3. Have you ever been taking:
   - Antibiotics, especially broad spectrum (Ampicillin, Bactrim, Keflex...)?
   - Tetracyclines for treatment for acne?
   - Birth control pills?
   - Cortisone, orally or in the form of injection (intra-muscular or intra-articular)
   - Immunosuppressive medications?

	YES	NO

4. Have you been living, or are you now in
   - Damp climates?
   - Moldy house?
   - Neighborhood of foggy beaches?

5. Have you been or are you an alcohol abuser?
   Have you been or are you using marihuana, cocaine or heroine?
   Do you smoke?

6. Have you had recurrent viral or bacterial infections?

7. Do you have an increased intake of raw food (salad bars)?

8. Have you had recurrent yeast infections (vaginal or nail)?

B. PRESENT HISTORY

9. Are your symptoms worse
   - on foggy, damp days?
   - when you are exposed to hay?
   - when you rake dry leaves?
   - when you are near a lawn that's being mowed?
   - when you are in a damp basement?

10. Are you craving for:
    - Sugar?
    - Breads?
    - Alcohol?

11. Do you feel increasingly more uncomfortable with your environment? (reacting to smoke, fumes, perfumes, pesticides, inability to visit public places)?

12. Are you allergic to Penicillin?

C. GASTROINTESTINAL SYMPTOMS

Are the following symptoms present?
   - Gas

	YES	NO

- Abdominal distention
- Diarrhea
- Constipation
- Hemorrhoids
- Abdominal pain
- Anal itching
- Mucus in stools
- Heartburn
- Indigestion
- Bad breath
- Aphthosis
- Constant hungry feeling
- Food allergies
- Weight loss or gain without change of diet
- Do you have a thick white or yellow fur in the middle of your tongue, especially in the morning?

D. BRAIN SYMPTOMS

Are the following symptoms present?

- Difficulties in concentration
- Decreased attention span
- Decreased memory
- Fogginess in the brain
- Drowsiness
- Incoordination
- Headaches
- Severe mood swings
- Depression
- Suicidal thoughts
- Anger and irritability
- Frustration
- Being defensive, even when it is not needed

E. HORMONAL SYMPTOMS

Are the following symptoms present?

- PMS
- Flare-up of yeast infections the week before the cycle

	YES	NO

- Loss of sexual desire
- Impotence
- Endometriosis
- Menstrual irregularities
- Flare-up of yeast infections after sexual intercourse

F. OTHER SYMPTOMS

- Tightness in the chest
- Palpitations
- Urgency, frequency and burning in the urination
- Postnasal drip
- Muscle pains, especially in the neck region
- Joint pains
- Feeling hot inside while cold on the outside
- Cold hands and feet
- Water retention
- Your doctor told you it is all "in your head"
- Your doctor told you it is "psychosomatic"
- Social isolation because of the "allergies" to food, smoke, fumes and disbelief of your friends
- Prostatitis
- Difficulties swallowing
- Sore throat
- Burning of the eyelids
- Itchy scaling skin lesions

All of these symptoms can be present in a thousand diseases. However, it is the simultaneous presence of the majority of the above complaints that is so specific for the Candida Syndrome.

APPENDIX II: HEALTH FOOD STORES AND SELECTED RESTAURANTS IN SOUTHERN CALIFORNIA

EREWHON
8001 Beverly Boulevard
Los Angeles, CA
(213) 655-5441

LICATA'S CALIFORNIA NUTRITION CENTERS
18538 Beach Boulevard
Huntington Beach, CA
(714) 962-9712

FULL OF LIFE, INC.
2515 W. Magnolia Boulevard
Burbank, CA

LINDBERG NUTRITION
6603 Fallbrook Avenue
Canoga Park, CA
(213) 348-5123

PLEASANT HOUSE OF NATURAL FOODS, INC.
535 "I" Street
Chula Vista, CA
(619) 427-7673

QUINN'S NUTRITION CENTER
11251 National Boulevard
Los Angeles, CA 90064

QUINN'S NUTRITION CENTERS
1864 N. Vermont Avenue
Los Angeles, CA 90027

QUINN'S NUTRITION CENTERS
8466 Melrose Avenue
Los Angeles, CA 90069

QUINN'S NUTRITION CENTERS
227 N. Larchmont Boulevard
Los Angeles,CA 90004

WEIDNER'S NUTRITION CENTERS
820 E. Colorado Boulevard
Pasadena, CA 91101
(818) 792-3189

CAMPBELL'S NUTRITION
Heisun Chung
928 Montana Avenue
Santa Monica, CA 90403

SELECTED RESTAURANTS

FOLLOW YOUR HEART
   21825 Sherman Way
   Canoga Park   (213) 348-3240

THE GOOD EARTH RESTAURANT
   17212 Ventura Boulevard
   Encino   (619) 986-9990

THE ARTFUL BALANCE
   525 1/2 North Fairfax Avenue
   Los Angeles   (213) 852-9091

EAST WEST FAMILY KITCHEN
   706 North Orange Grove Avenue
   Los Angeles   (213) 852-9587

EREWHON NATURAL FOODS
   8001 Beverly Boulevard
   Los Angeles   (213) 655-5441

GOLDEN CARROTS
   8849 Sunset Boulevard
   Los Angeles   (213) 659-3380

GRAIN COUNTRY
   7827 Melrose
   Los Angeles   (213) 655-3948

INAKA NATURAL FOOD RESTAURANT
   131 South La Brea
   Los Angeles   (213) 932-8869

SUNFLOWER CAFE
   8639 Lincoln Boulevard
   Los Angeles   (213) 641-2113

WHITE MEMORIAL MEDICAL CENTER CAFETERIA
   1720 Brooklyn Avenue
   Los Angeles   (213) 268-5000

MOTHER NATURE'S
   5424 Laurel Canyon Avenue
   North Hollywood (213) 985-2163

ACCENT ON HEALTH
   18531 Devonshire Street
   Northridge   (213) 360-1516

ONE LIFE NATURAL FOODS
   3001 Main Street
   Santa Monica   (213) 392-4501

INN OF THE 7th RAY
    128 Old Topanga Canyon Road
    Topanga   (213) 455-1311

SUN VITAMINS
    17228 Hawthorne Boulevard
    Torrance   (213) 371-4844

THE COMEBACK INN
    1633 West Washington Boulevard
    Venice   (213) 396-7255

FULL CIRCLE WHOLE FOODS
    425 Ocean Front Walk
    Venice   (213) 399-2390

THE GOOD EARTH RESTAURANT
    1002 Westwood Boulevard
    Westwood   (213) 208-0215

OLD WORLD RESTAURANT
    1019 Westwood Boulevard
    Westwood   (213) 208-4033

THE GOOD EARTH RESTAURANT
    23397 Mulholland Drive
    Woodland Hills (213) 888-6300

The above named restaurants are the best choices for Candida patients. None of the foods presented contain preservatives, artificial flavors or colors. Add to these restaurants most Chinese ones (omit the MSG!), some Japanese ones (omit the Sushi!) and Thai restaurants.

APPENDIX III: CANDIDA SUPPORT GROUPS AND OTHER SOURCES OF HELP.

1. Candida Research and Information Foundation (Support Group)
P.O. Box 2719
Castro Valley, CA 94546
(415) 582-2179
Person in charge: Gayle Nielsen

2. L.A. Center (Support Group)
1703 Wilshire Boulevard
Santa Monica, CA 90403
(213) 453-4565
Person in charge: Carol Skegas
When: Saturdays, 1 p.m.
Enrollment limited
Pre-registration necessary.

3. GRL Inc.
8900 Winnetka Avenue
Winnetka, CA 91324-3243
(818) 349-9911
For "Celginate", Lactobacillus liquid, Zinc Orothate,
Hemolin, Beta Carotene, Selenium (Algasel), Vitamin E,
Capryllin and Polyzym O-22.

4. Natren
10935 Camarillo Street
No. Hollywood, CA 91602
(818) 766-9300, (818) 769-9300
For Megadophilus (Superdophilus) and Bifido.

5. Creative Living Center (Counselors)
Joe L. McNair, Ph.D.
Director
4525 Sherman Oaks Avenue
Sherman Oaks, CA 91403
(213) 990-9900

6. Family Counseling West (Counselors)
21921 Viscanio Road
Woodland Hills, CA 91364
(818) 999-6164
With branches in Sherman Oaks, Granada Hills, Westlake,
West Los Angeles (213/474-2151)

7. Jordan and Margaret Paul, Ph.D's (Counselors)
3127 Corinth Avenue
Los Angeles, CA 90066
(213) 390-5993

8. Kyolic
   Wakunaga of America Co. Ltd.
   23501 Madero
   Mission Viejo, CA   92691
   (800) 544-5800

9. Ms. Gloria Axelrod, Ed.M.
   931 Gayley Avenue
   Los Angeles, CA   90024
   (213) 208-8729
   Communications consultant, individual and group sessions.

APPENDIX IV: THE MOST COMMON AND PRACTICAL TREATMENT PLAN FOR THE CANDIDA PATIENT.

WEEK 1:
- The anti-yeast diet
- Lactobacillus liquid, 1 Tbs. three times a day after meals or Megadophilus powder, 1 tsp., three times a day, between meals.
- Pau D'Arco tea or Taheebo tea: 2 cups a day, add cinnamon or lemon, if desired.
- Garlic (Kyolic), 6 capsules a day (2/2/2), with meals.
- Biotin 5 mg, 1 a day.
- Celginate 3+3+3 with meals, if constipated.

WEEK 2:

Add to the above products:
- Capryllin capsules in an increasing dose:

  Day 1:   1/1/1 (1 capsule WITH each meal, 1-2 if only 2 meals)

  Day 2:   2/2/2

  Day 3-7: 3/3/3

  Day 8-16: 4/4/4

  Day 17:   2 and 2 (4 in total), for 1 month.

Take Capryllin always WITH meals.

If necessary, the maintenance dose (4), can be continued for 2 more months. Not longer, since the patient probably did not stick to a good diet plan.

WEEK 5: (at this moment, we are on 2/2 Capryllin):
1. Stick to the program of Week 1
2. You may start adding some foods:
   - yeast-free rye or wheat breads (in health foods stores)
   - maple syrup or some honey
   - some more fruits (no apples-pears or grapes); try cantelope, peaches (without peels), all berries; do not add any other food with this fruit, eat it as a breakfast.

3. Boost your immune system in order to avoid relapses:
    - Vitamin C: 4000-10,000 mgs. daily (up to bowel tolerance)
    - Vitamin E: 400 U.I. daily, combined with 100 mcg. Selenium, Zinc orothate, 50 mgs. daily
    - Polyzym 0 22: 10 daily between meals
    - Evening Primrose Oil: 4 capsules daily (each at least 40 mgs. GLA)

It is advisable to boost your immune system for at least 3 months (if not for the rest of your life!).

After three months on this program, the patient should be able to eat most of the foods. It does not mean that this is the moment to become a sugar-alcoholic. Cravings will not be a problem any more.

From Week 1 on: ACUPUNCTURE treatments, to increase the energy in the Spleen-Pancreas (and boost the immune system): once a week for 4 weeks. From Week 5 on: once every 14 days for 1 month. Then, once every 3 weeks for 2 months.

This treatment plan is convenient and helpful for most of the patients. However, the patient needs to be followed by a holistic, nutritional oriented M.D.

APPENDIX V: FOOD RECIPES

A. BREAKFAST

- Ricecakes
- Eggs
- Brown Rice Cream
- "Rice and Shine" cereal by Arrowhead

- Tropical fruits
- Brown Rice Bran
- Amaranth cereal
- Quinoa

<u>Bread Recipes:</u>

CANDIDA BREAD
(Phil Gernhard)

1 1/4 cups brown rice flour
2 eggs
1 1/2 cups grated carrots or banana
3/4 cup safflower oil or 3/4 cup butter
1 tsp. baking soda
1 tsp. baking powder
1/4 tsp. nutmeg
1/4 tsp. cinnamon
1/2 tsp. vanilla or other extract
3 tbs. yogurt

Mix all together.

Bake one hour at 325 in a preheated oven.

BANANA RICE BREAD

2 cups brown rice flour
1/2 cup corn flour
3 tsp. baking powder
1/4 tsp. sea salt (optional)
1/2 cup melted butter
1 1/2 cups mashed bananas
2/3 cup corn syrup
2 eggs

Stir flour, baking powder, salt together.

In a separate bowl, beat the butter and corn syrup together, add eggs, beat and add the bananas, beat well; then add the dry mixture, mx well. Pour into a small well greased loaf pan.

Bake at 350 degrees for about 1/2 hour or until a toothpick stuck in the center comes out dry. Do not overbake.

CORN BREAD

1 1/2 cups corn flour
1/2 cup brown rice flour
3 tsp. baking powder
1/4 tsp. sea salt (optional)
3 tbs. corn syrup
1 cup goats milk or soya milk
1/4 cup vegetable oil

Mix the dry ingredients together.

In a separate bowl, beat the liquids together; add the dry mixture to the liquid, mix well. Pour into a small well greased baking dish. Bake at 350 degrees for 25-30 minutes or until a toothpick stuck in the center comes out dry. Do not overbake.

NON YEAST RICE CARROT BREAD

2 1/2 cups brown rice flour
1/4 tsp. salt (optional)
3 tbs. baking powder
1 level tsp. baking soda
2 eggs
3 tbs. honey
5 tbs. lemon juice
1/4 cup chopped carrots
1/4 cup walnuts, crushed
1 cup raisins
1/2 cup butter or oleo

Mix the powders together in a bowl.

In a blender, add the butter, eggs and milk. Start blender at blender speed, add the carrots slowly until blended. Pour into a separate bowl, mix in the walnuts, raisins and lemon juice. Mix well. Add the mixed flour powder into the bowl and mix well.

Pour into a well greased baking dish, tap dish on counter top 2 or 3 times, set into oven at 350 degrees. Bake for 25 to 30 minutes or until a thin sharp knife inserted in the center comes out dry. Do not overbake.

AMARANTH PANCAKES/FLATBREAD

1/2 cup almond nuts, ground
1 cup amaranth flour
1/2 cup arrowroot
1 tsp. baking soda
1/4 tsp. sea salt
1 tsp. cinnamon
1 1/4 cups water
2 tbs. lemon juice
2 tbs. oil

Grind nuts in blender about 15 seconds. Combine with other dry ingredients in mixing bowl. Without washing it, combine liquids in blender; blend 10 seconds and stir into dry mixture. Cook pancakes on preheated, ungreased non-stick frypan. When bubbly and brown, turn. As batter thickens, you may need to add another tbs. or two of water to keep cakes thin.

If you want to use pancakes as flatbread, remove to wire racks to cool. When cool, stack, wrap and refrigerate. May toast in toaster oven or place on wire racks on cookie sheets in moderate oven for a few minutes. Make mini sandwiches; try sliced chicken or turkey, garnished with lettuce and tomato.

AMARANTH BANANA BREAD

1/4 cup nuts, finely ground
1 3/4 cups sifted rice flour + 1/2 cup sifted amaranth
    OR 1 3/4 cups sifted amaranth flour + 1/2 cup arrowroot
1/2 tsp. sea salt
2 tsp. baking soda
1/2 cup nuts, coarsely chopped
1 1/2 cups very ripe banana, mashed (2 cups of 1" pieces)
2 tbs. lemon juice
1/4 cup oil
2 eggs
1 teaspoon vanilla

Preheat oven to 350 degrees. Grease on 9" x 5" pan or two 7" x 3". Grind nuts in blender. Add to remaining dry ingredients in large mixing bowl, and add coarse nuts. Without washing equipment, combine remaining ingredients in blender and process 30 seconds. Pour liquids over dry mixture and stir, but do not beat.

Pour into prepared pan(s) and bake large loaf 55-60 minutes; or about 45 minutes for small loaves. Bread is done when toothpick inserted in center comes out clean and dry. After 10 minutes at room temperature, turn loaves out on wire rack to cool.

RICE PANCAKES

1 egg
1 cup goats milk
2 tbs. sunflower seed oil
1 cup rice flour
1 tsp. baking powder
1/2 tsp. soda
1/2 tsp. salt (optional)

Beat egg; add remaining ingredients in order listed and best with rotary beater until smooth. Grease heated griddle if necessary. To test griddle, sprinkle with few drops of water. If bubbles skitter around, heat is just right.

Pour batter from tip of large spoon or from pitcher onto hot griddle. Turn pancakes as soon as they are puffed and full of bubbles but before bubbles break. Bake other side until golden brown.

GINGERBREAD

1 1/2 cups amaranth flour AND 1/2 cup arrowroot
OR 1 1/2 cups brown rice flour AND 1/2 cup amaranth flour
1 teaspoon baking soda
3/4 tsp. ginger
1 tsp. cinnamon
1/4 tsp. allspice
2/3 cup warm water
1/4 cup oil
2 tbs. lemon juice

Grease 9 inch baking dish. Preheat oven to 350 degrees. Combine dry ingredients and sift them into bowl, mixing them well. Combine liquids in one pint measuring cup and mix with fork. Pour over dry ingredients all at once and mix quickly.

Pour immediately into prepared baking dish. Bake 30 minutes. When done, cracks appear and top springs back when touched. Serve warm.

NUT 'N SEED CRUNCH CRUST

1/2 cup flour - brown rice or amaranth
1 tbs. arrowroot
1/2 cup ground nuts (except peanuts)
1/4 cup sunflower seeds
1/2 tsp. cinnamon
1/8 tsp. cloves
2 tbs. oil
2 tbs. water

Combine dry ingredients in small bowl. Put oil in small sauce pan and heat gently. Pour the liquid over the dry ingredients and mix with fork. Press into oiled pie pan. Bake at 350 degrees for 10 minutes if filling with pumpkin or other filling that has to bake. Excellent flavor with crunch.

PINEAPPLE PRUNE CAKE

1 cup pitted prunes
8 oz. fresh crushed pineapple in its own juice
1 6 oz. can frozen pineapple juice concentrate
1 tsp. cinnamon
1/4 tsp. cloves
1/4 cup vegetable oil
1 1/4 cup amaranth flour
1/2 cup arrowroot powder
1 1/2 tsp. baking soda
1 cup nuts (no peanuts)
2 large eggs
1 tsp. vanilla

Measure 1/2 cup of juice concentrate for cake; reserve remaining 1/4 cup for glaze.

Chop prunes; mix with undrained pineapple and juice concentrate in a 2 or 3 quart saucepan. Add spices. Bring fruit to boil and simmer 5 minutes; set aside to cool. Stir in oil. In separate bowl, combine dry ingredients and mix them thoroughly. Grease a 9" x 9" glass baking dish. When fruit mixture is lukewarm, add eggs and vanilla and beat with wooden spoon for 2 minutes. Add dry ingredients and stir until they disappear. Pour batter into prepared baking dish. Bake at 350 degrees for 35-40 minutes.

Make glaze when cake is removed from oven.

CAROB FUDGE CAKE

1 1/8 cup sifted amaranth flour AND 1/2 cup arrowroot
OR 1 cup sifted brown rice flour AND 1/2 cup sifted amaranth
flour
1/4 cup carob powder
1 tsp. baking soda
2/3 cup warm water
1/3 cup oil
1 tbs. vanilla
1/4 cup chopped nuts

Grease 9" baking dish. Preheat oven to 350 degrees.

Combine dry ingredients and sift them into bowl, mixing them
well. Combine liquids in one pint measuring cup and mix them
with fork. Pour over dry ingredients all at once and mix
quickly.

Pour immediately into prepared baking dish. Scatter nuts on
top of batter. Bake 25-30 minutes. Typically, cracks appear
in top when done. Inside remains moist and fudgy. Best
served warm or within a day.

BROWNIES

Follow Carob Fudge Cake recipe exactly, except reduce water
to 1/4 cup. Batter will be thick; spread thinly in a greased
11" x 7" x 12" pan. Bake at 350 degrees for 20-25 minutes.

BASIC COOKIE BATTER

3 tbs. oil
3 tbs. water
1 cup amaranth flour
1/3 cup arrowroot
1/2 tsp. baking soda
1/4 tsp. salt
1/8 tsp. vitamin C crystals
1 tsp. vanilla

Combine oil and water in saucepan. Heat gently and remove
from heat to cool. Sift flours before measuring. Combine
dry ingredients and sift again. Stir vanilla into liquids,
then add dry ingredients. Add any additional ingredients you
choose. Drop batter by rounded teaspoon onto cookie sheet.
Bake 12-15 minutes, until cookies are brown. Remove to wire
rack to cool. Yields about 2 dozen.

CHIPPIES

1/3 cup carob chips
1/3 cup chopped nuts

Add to BASIC COOKIE BATTER

CARROT COOKIES

3/4 cup grated carrot
1/3 cup raisins
1/2 tsp. cinnamon

Add to BASIC COOKIE BATTER

SPICY GINGER GEMS

1/2 tsp. ginger
1/2 tsp. cinnamon
1/4 tsp. allspice

Sift spices with dry ingredients. May omit vanilla. Proceed
as directed.

FUDGIES

IN PLACE OF ARROWROOT use 1/3 cup sifted carob powder.
Optional: 1/3 cup chopped nuts may be added or each FUDGIE
may be topped with half a nut. Proceed as directed.

PIE CRUST

3/4 cup amaranth flour
1/2 cup arrowroot
1/4 cup nuts, seeds or peanuts, finely ground
1/4 tsp. salt
1/2 tsp. cinnamon, optional
3 tbs. oil
3 to 4 tbs. water

Combine dry ingredients and blend well. Combine oil and 3
tablespoons water, and blend with fork. Add all at once to
flour. Stir only until a ball forms. If ball appears dry
and crumbly, add a little more water, one teaspoon at a time,
until ball hangs together. (Moisture content of flour
varies). Oil 9" pie plat, or use oil and liquid lecithin.
Pat or roll crust to fit. Dough tears easily, but mends
easily using extra bits to patch. Prick with fork. Bake 3
minutes at 400 degrees, fill and finish baking the time
required for filling. Or, bake about 15 minutes until brown
and crisp. Cool and fill. Crust holds up very well after
baking.

SAVORY CRACKERS

1 recipe PIE CRUST dough
1/2 tsp. baking soda
1/8 tsp. vitamin C crystals
Optional Seasonings: 1/2 tsp. caraway seeds, OR 1/2 tsp. chili powder, OR 1/4 tsp. onion powder + 1/8 tsp. garlic powder, OR 1 tsp. herbs of your choice (oregano, basil, tarragon, etc.)
Sesame seeds

Combine soda, Vitamin C and seasonings with other dry ingredients. Mix as directed. Scatter sesame seeds directly on cookie sheet. Roll half of dough at a time, rolling quite thin, 1/8 to 1/4 inch. Cut into 1 1/2" squares or triangles, prick with fork and bake 15 minutes at 350 degrees. Separate crackers and place on wire racks. Place wire rack on cookie sheet and return to oven to crisp another 5 to 7 minutes. Cool completely before storing in airtight container. Repeat with other half of dough. For a saltine-type cracker, sprinkle unbaked crackers VERY LIGHTLY with salt. Yields 3 or 4 dozen.

QUINOA (THE BASIC RECIPE)

2 cups water
1 cup quinoa

Rinse quinoa thoroughly, either by using a strainer or by running fresh water over the quinoa in a pot. Drain excess water. Place quinoa and water in a 1 1/2 quart saucepan and bring to a boil. Reduce to a simmer, cover, and cook until all of the water is absorbed (10-15 minutes). You will know that the quinoa is done when all the grains have turned from white to transparent. Yields: 4 cups

QUINOA (WITH A GOURMET TOUCH)

4 cups water
1/8 to 1/4 tsp. sea salt
2 cups quinoa

Place water and salt in a 2 quart saucepan and bring to a rapid boil. While water is heating, place quinoa in a wok or thin steel pan (cast iron is not advised) and, while stirring continuously with a wooden spoon, toast for about 10 minutes or until the color is a shade deeper and the quinoa emits a delicate fragrance. Add toasted quinoa to boiling water, cover, reduce to a simmer and cook until all of the water is absorbed (15-20 minutes). Remove from fire and allow to sit for 5 to 10 minutes. With a damp wooden spook, mix quinoa in the pot. Cover and allow to rest for another 5 to 10 minutes. Place in a wooden serving bowl and serve. Yields: 8 cups

Variations: For a richer, nutty flavor, toast quinoa in 1 tsp. unrefined oil. For a heartier flavor, saute a pressed garlic clove and then toast the quinoa. Substitute 1 tsp. natural shoyu for the sea salt.

BUCKWHEAT AND QUINOA

4 cups water
1/8 to 1/4 tsp. sea salt
1 cup unroasted buckwheat
1 cup quinoa

Place the water and salt in a 1 1/2 quart saucepan and bring to a boil. While water is heating, place buckwheat in a wok or skillet and toast over a high flame, while stirring constantly, until it turns an amber color and emits a deep aroma. Set aside. Toast the quinoa until it turns a shade darker in color, about 10 minutes.

When the water is boiling add quinoa first and then 'slowly' add the buckwheat or the water will bubble over the pot. Reduce the fire to low, cover and allow to simmer until all of the water is absorbed (15-20 minutes). Remove from heat and allow to rest for 5 to 10 minutes. With a damp wooden spoon, gently mix the grain from top to bottom while still in the pot. Cover again and allow to set for 5 to 10 minutes. Place in a serving bowl (preferably wooden) and serve.

THE ULTIMATE DRINK
(Betty Endicott)

Papaya (1 large size glass)
Yolk of a fertile egg
1 banana
1/2 cup tofu, cut small
1/4 cup brown rice

Put all the ingredients together in a blender and enjoy this thick, nutritious mixture.

CARROT MUFFINS

1 cup rice flour
1 1/2 tsp. baking powder
1 egg
1/2 cup fresh carrot juice
1 carrot, grated
2 1/2 tbs. butter, melted

Preheat over to 400. Mix together flour and baking powder. Beat egg, add juice, carrot and butter. Pour into flour mixture. Stir until just mixed but still somewhat lumpy. Divide batter evenly into 8 muffin cups, 1/2 full. Bake for 30 minutes.

CORN RICE MUFFINS

1 1/3 brown rice flour
1/2 cup yellow corn flour
5 tsp. baking powder
2 eggs (divided)
1/4 cup Amazake
1/2 cup and 2 tbs. water
1 34/ tbs. melted butter

Mix dry ingredients. Beat egg yolk and add Amazake, water and butter. Blend with dry ingredients using gentle strokes. Beat egg whites stiff and fold gently into batter. Fill muffin cups, 1/2 full. Bake at 375 degrees for 25 minutes.

B. LUNCH AND DINNER

LEMON BUTTER SAUCE

1/3 cup butter
Dash pepper, to taste
1/4 cup lemon juice
2 tbs. finely chopped parsley

Melt butter in small saucepan over low heat. Add pepper, lemon juice and parsley. Cook till everything is well-heated. Serve at once. Makes about 1/2 cup sauce.

ASPARAGUS

1/4 cup olive oil
1 onion, thinly sliced
1/2 green pepper, deseeded and chopped
1 8-oz. can tomatoes, drained (but reserve liquid)
1/2 cup chopped celery
1/4 cup juice from tomatoes
1/4 cup chopped parsley
Salt and pepper, to taste
1 lb. fresh asparagus

Heat oil in large saucepan. Saute the onion and green pepper till tender. Add tomatoes, celery, juice, parsley and salt and pepper. Add asparagus and cook till asparagus is tender. Serves 5-6.

SWEET POTATO JUMBLE

1 lb. sweet potatoes
1 tbs. sesame seeds
3 tbs. miso (red or dark)
1/4 cup stock

Peel the sweet potatoes and cut in 1/2 inch dice. Steam or simmer until just tender. Set aside.

Heat the sesame seeds in a non-stick pan until they begin to jump. Remove from the pan immediately. Crush or grind them while hot.*

Mix the crushed seeds with the mso and stock. Stir in the potatoes.

Cook over low heat about 5 minutes to blend the flavors. (A non-stick pan is best.)

Serve hot or cold as a side dish or rice topping. Serves 4.
Suggestions: Garnish with minced scallion, toasted sesame
seeds or both.

*If possible, use a ridged Japanese grinding bowl called a
suribachi.

EASY SOUP

4 cups sliced vegetables, such as onions, red bell pepper,
tomatoes, corn, celery, spinach, squash, etc.
2 tbs. minced parsley
4 cups good vegetable or chicken broth (look for canned or
packaged bouillon in the natural foods store, or make your
own)
2 tbs. light miso blended with 4 tbs. hot water
Herbal salt and pepper, to taste
1 cooked potato, chopped in small pieces

VEGGIE STIR FRY

1/2 onion, chopped
2 stalks celery, thinly sliced
1/2 head cauliflower, chopped
1/2 head broccoli, chopped
1 carrot, pared into curls
1 green pepper, chopped (or thin sliced)
2 cups snow peas
1-2 cups fresh mushrooms, sliced
Dash low sodium soy sauce
Dash fresh ginger, grated
1-2 cloves garlic, finely minced
2 tbs. oil

Wash and prepare all vegetables. Heat oil in skillet. Saute
onion, garlic, celery, cauliflower, broccoli and green
pepper. When still crisp, add carrot curls, snow peas, fresh
mushrooms, soy sauce and ginger. Continue to cook till all
vegetables are crisp cooked. Serve at once. Serves 3-4.

WINTER LENTIL SOUP

1 cup lentils
1 1/2 cup water
1 medium potato
1 small turnip
1 small carrot
1 medium diced onion
1 clove crushed garlic
1/4 tsp. thyme
3 tbs. soy sauce
Salt and pepper, to taste

Cook lentils in water, covered for 25-30 minutes until tender but not mushy.

Meanwhile, dice potato, turnip and carrot. If they are organically grown and not paraffinned, don't peel them. Put them in a pot with water to cover, cook about 10 minutes or until just tender.

Add lentils and their cooking water, if any, to diced vegetables and their cooking water. Add everything else and as much water as you like to make a fairly thick soup.

SEA STEAKS WITH ALMONDS

4 medium sized fish fillets, rather thin
1 tbs. oil
1 tbs. butter
4 large scallions, chopped
1/2 cup sliced fresh almonds
4 tbs. lemon juice
4 tbs. Worcestershire sauce
Freshly ground pepper
Dash cayenne

Wash fish and dry thoroughly. Heat oil and butter rather hot. Fry fish until brown on one side. Turn and cook on other side. When fish is almost done, add scallions. Cook a few minutes, then add mushrooms. Cook a few minutes more. Season with lemon juice, Worcestershire sauce, freshly ground pepper and a dash of cayenne. Serve hot. Serves 4.

LENTILS WITH SPINACH

4 tbs. butter
1 cup rice, rinsed
6 cups boiling water
1 tsp. salt
1 cup lentils, rinsed
4 tbs. olive oil
10 oz. fresh spinach, thoroughly washed and chopped
4 cloves garlic, crushed
1/4 cup finely chopped fresh coriander leaves
1/2 tsp. pepper
1/2 tsp. cumin
1 tsp. oregano
tsp. sumac (a powdered spice found in Middle Eastern markets
 - optional)

In a frying pan, melt the butter, then stir-fry the rice over high heat for 3 minutes.

Add 2 cups of the water and bring to a boil, then stir in 1/2 tsp. of the salt. Cover and turn the heat to low.

Cook for 15 minutes, then turn the heat off and allow to cook in its own steam for 20 minutes. Set aside.

In the meantime, in a saucepan, place the lentils and the remaining 4 cups of water and bring to a boil. Cover and cook over medium heat for 30 minutes or until the lentils are cooked but not mushy. Drain and set aside.

In another frying pan, heat the oil. Add the spinach and garlic and saute over medium heat until the spinach wilts.

Add the lentils, remaining salt, coriander leaves, pepper, cumin and oregano, then saute for a further 8 minutes, stirring once in a while.

Place the frying plan contents on a flat serving platter, then spread the rice evenly over the top. Sprinkle with the sumac just before serving. Serve hot. Serves 8 to 10.

BEAN AND LENTIL STEW

1/2 cup navy beans, soaked overnight and drained
9 cups water
1 cup lentils, rinsed
4 tsp. olive oil
2 medium-sized onions, chopped
4 cloves garlic, crushed
1 hot pepper, finely chopped
1/4 cup rise, rinsed
1 tsp. cumin
1 tsp. oregano
1 tsp. salt
1/2 tsp. pepper
3 tbs. very finely chopped fresh coriander leaves

In a saucepan, place the beans and water and bring to a boil, then cover and cook over medium heat for 1 1/4 hours.

Add the lentils and cook for a further 20 minutes.

In the meantime, in a frying pan, heat the oil, then saute the onions until they turn golden brown.

Add the garlic and hot pepper, and stir-fry for an additional 3 minutes.

Add the frying plan contents and the remaining ingredients (except the coriander leaves) to the lentils and beans, then cover and simmer over low heat for 30 minutes or until the lentils and beans are cooked. Stir once in a while to make sure the stew does not stick to the bottom of the pot.

Stir in the coriander leaves and serve hot. Serves 6 to 8.

SWEET PEPPERS WITH BASIL

4 tbsp. olive or vegetable oil
1 medium-sized onion, chopped
2 cloves garlic, crushed
4 large sweet red peppers, seeded and chopped
1 tsp. oregano
1/2 tsp. sea salt
1/4 tsp. pepper
4 tbs. finely chopped fresh basil or tsp. dried
2 tbs. lemon juice

In a frying pan, heat the oil, then stir-fry the onion and garlic until the onion turns limp.

Stir in the pepper pieces, oregano, salt and pepper, then saute over medium heat for about 15 minutes or until the pepper pieces turn limp, stirring occasionally.

Stir in the basil and lemon juice. Serve immediately. Serves 4.

HERBED FISH AND RICE

2 tbs. oil
1 cup raw brown rice
3 tbs. chopped onion
Salt and pepper
2 tbs. salt-free Italian
    herb seasoning
2 cups water
3 tbs. fresh parsley, chopped

2 cups frozen peas
4 medium cod fillets
Lemon juice
Paprika
1 tbs. butter
1 cup chicken broth
1/2 tsp. curry powder

In a medium sized saucepan, heat the oil and cook the rice and onion in it for a few minutes to toast the rice. Add the salt and pepper, the herb seasoning and the water. Bring water to a boil, turn to a low heat and cook 45 minutes until all water is absorbed. Cool. Add the chopped fresh parsley. Refrigerate until needed. At cooking time, oil large casserole dish. Rinse frozen peas in lukewarm water and drain. Alternate in casserole dish with the rice. Wash fish fillets and season with lemon juice, salt and pepper. Arrange on top of the rice, sprinkle with paprika, dot with butter and garnish with lemon peel strips. Mix chicken broth with curry powder. Pour around sides of casserole. Dot peas with butter. Cover casserole and bake at 350 for 30 minutes, covered. Uncover and bake 10 minutes more. Very elegant and mild tasting. Serves 4.

LAMB CHOPS WITH BASIL SAUCE

2 tbs. olive oil
8 lamb chops
1 tsp. salt
1 tsp. thyme
1/4 tsp. pepper
1/8 tsp. cayenne
1 medium-sized onion, finely chopped
2 cloves garlic, crushed
1 1/2 tbs. flour
1 cup water
2 tsp. dried basil, or 2 tbs. fresh, chopped

In a frying pan, heat the oil, then add the lamb chops and sprinkle with thyme, pepper, cayenne and 1/2 teaspoon of the salt.

Saute over medium heat, turning the chops over a few times until they are well done. Remove the chops and place on a serving platter.

If there is too much fat in the frying pan, remove a little, then add the onion and garlic and saute until the onion pieces turn golden brown.

Add the flour and stir-fry for 2 minutes, then stir in the water and remaining 1/2 tsp. of salt. Simmer for about 2 minutes, stirring all the time.

Stir in the basil, then pour evenly over the chops and serve immediately with mashed potatoes. Serves 4.

TOFU STIR FRY

1 onion or 2 leeks (sliced)
2-3 cloves garlic (minced)
1 pkg. tofu (drained and cubed)

Put in a wok and saute in 1 tbs. sesame oil and a few squirts.

ADD: carrot and parsnip spears
        broccoli flowerettes and sliced stems
        chinese cabbage
        chopped parsley
        imitation chicken broth
        Bragg's liquid aminos
        Wachters Sea and Land seasoning
        1/2 - 1 tsp. arrowroot or cornstarch (dissolved in
            water)

Do not overcook! Vegetables should be tender crisp. Serve with brown rice or other grain.

TOFU 'CHEESE' SAUCE

2-3 green onions
2-3 cloves garlic
1 tbs. corn oil
1 pkg. tofu, drained and <u>steamed</u>
4 umeboshi plums, pits removed (or 4 tsp. umeboshi paste)
1/2" slice Nuka (pickled daikon)
1 tbs. miso (mellow white)

Fresh herb of choice (e.g. basil, dill or whatever you like)
Optional: carrots, red bell pepper, extra onion.

Saute onion and gaelic in oil until slightly brown. Add any
other vegetables and cook for a few minutes longer. Process
or blend <u>steamed</u> tofu and all other ingredients until smooth.
use think to put in omelettes or casseroles, or thin with
water and serve hot over Japanese buckwheat noodles.

TOFUNAISE

1 pkg. tofu
1-2 cloves garlic, minced
Fresh dill, minced or dried dill
1 tbs. miso (mellow white) OR Bragg's liquid aminos OR sea
  salt
1 tbs. fresh lemon juice

While food processor is running, drop in garlic and fresh
herbs to mince. Add rest of ingredients and blend smooth.
Variation: Try curry instead of dill to season.

May be used as a dip for chips or vegetables, as well as a
substitute for mayonnaise.

NON-DAIRY TOFU DIP

Combine "Miso + Plus Mix" (Chive Dip Mix) with 8 oz. tofu, 3
tbs. tahini, 1 oz. (1/8 cup) water and 1 tsp. lemon juice in
a blender or food processor. Blend thoroughly and chill 1
hour before serving. Optional: 1-2 tbs. Hain natural kosher
dill relish (contains no vinegar).

Serve with chips, crackers or vegetables.

CACTUS COLLAGE

2-3 green onions, chopped
2 cloves garlic, chopped
1 pc. napal cactus - use potato peeler to remove base of
    stickers
1 tbs. oil
Several stalks bok choy, sliced
Mung bean sprouts, rinsed
1/3 cup parsley (fresh), chopped
Fresh tarragon or dried
Bragg's liquid aminos OR salt and pepper

Saute onions and garlic in oil. Cut cactus in small squares
and add. Add the rest of the ingredients. Season to taste.
Serve with a grain. Serves 2-3.

SQUASH CASSEROLE

2 sm. or 1 very lg. butternut squash (cooked & mashed)
1/4 cup butter (divided: 3 tbs. & 1 tbs.)
1/2 - 1 tsp. salt (according to taste) OR 1/2 tsp. Bragg's
    liquid aminos
1/8 tsp. pepper
1 tsp. onion (minced)
3 eggs (well beaten) OR egg substitute
1/4 cup crispy brown rice cereal OR crushed tortilla chips OR
    crushed corn flakes OR crushed rice cake

Earlier in the day, cut butternut squash in 1/2 and scoop out
seeds. Place on edged cookie sheet - cut side down. Bake 45
minutes - 1 hour at 325 (until soft to the touch). Cool and
peel.

If you have a food processor, process onion first to mince.
Add eggs and process until well beaten. Add peeled, cooked
squash and process until smooth. Add 3 tbs. butter (melted),
seasoning and soy milk (if desired).

Pour into greased 1 1/2 qt. casserole dish. Top with
buttered brown rice crispies or crumbs of your (use remaining
1 tbs. butter).

Set in a pan of warm water and bake at 350 until knife
inserted in center comes out clean (45 mins. - 1 hr.) Makes
6 servings.

Note: You can cook beans early in the day if you like. Drain and pour immediately into very cold water to cool quickly (this stops cooking and helps them stay crisp). Drain, cover and refrigerate. Later reheat and season. 8 servings.

RATATOUILLE

1/4 cup oil
1/2 medium onion, thinly sliced
1 large green pepper, cut in strips
1 medium zucchini, thinly sliced
1/2 large (or 2 small) eggplant, diced
4-5 medium tomatoes, chunked
 OR 1 16 oz. can tomatoes
3/4 - 1 tsp. salt or liquid aminos
1/4 tsp. ground white pepper
Dash cayenne pepper
Dash marjoram leaves (or fresh)
2 cloves garlic, minced
2-4 tbs. fresh, chopped parsley

Heat olive oil in saucepan. Add onion and green pepper. Saute a few minutes until onion is wilted. Add rest of ingredients. Mix well and simmer over low heat 15-20 minutes, stirring occasionally, until vegetables are just done.

Serve over rice (brown or basmati). 4-5 servings.

NORTHWESTERN SALMON

1 half or whole salmon (4 to 6 lbs.)
1/2 cup of butter plus 12 small bits of butter to insert in
    slashes
1/4 cup flour (of choice)
3/4 cup chopped celery
3/4 cup chopped onion
1 large can stewed tomatoes (28 oz. size) (sugar free)
2 bay leaves
paprika

Cut slashed in each side of the fish and insert the small butter bits. Place salmon on a large enough piece of heavy-duty foil to wrap it for baking. In saucepan, melt 1/2 cup of butter. Stir in flour and brown slightly. Add chopped celery and onion. Then, add tomatoes and bay leaves. Season to taste with salt, pepper and paprika. Cook, stirring constantly until sauce is slightly thickened. Pour the sauce inside and over the fish. Wrap foil securely around fish and bake at 325 for 15 minutes per pound. Serves 6 to 8.

NON-DAIRY CREAM OF VEGETABLE SOUP

2 tbs. unrefined oil
1/2 cup rice flour
4 cups water
1/4 tsp. sea salt
1 tbs. unrefined oil
2 onions, sliced
3 stalks celery, sliced OR 1 cup vegetable of choice,
    chopped, e.g. broccoli
1 tbs. Bragg's liquid aminos, or to taste
White pepper, to taste
Optional: add garlic and saute with onion & vegetables

Heat 2 tbs. oil in large saucepan; add rice flour and saute.
Cool and add water and salt, then simmer for 30 minutes.

Heat a small skillet. Add 1 tbs. oil, onions (& maybe
garlic) and vegetables and saute. Add them to the soup.
Simmer 15 minutes more. Add liquid aminos and pepper, and
perhaps chopped parsley mixed in.

Garnish with chopped fresh parsley; another option for a
garnish is imitation bacon bits. Makes 4 cups.

NUT (or SEED) CHEESE

1 lb. almonds
4 scallions
2-3 cloves garlic
1 handful Italian parsley or cilantro
Fresh basil or tarragon, to taste
1 carrot
1/2 celery stalk + leaves
1/2 red bell pepper (optional)
Bragg's liquid aminos (to taste)

Soak nuts (or seeds) overnight in spring or distilled water.
Drain and put into juicer with screen removed and homogenizer
cover in place. Grind nuts to fine texture. Replace screen
and remove cover. Juice rest of ingredients into nut
mixture; stir and season with liquid aminos.

Transfer to ceramic or glass covered container and set out at
room temperature for 6-8 hours, then refrigerate. Must eat
now! (Can't cook with it, but can crumble over things. Try
sesame seeds and season with caraway seeds, as well as other
things.)

OTHER VEGETABLES:

cauliflower
zucchini
bok choy
celery
green or red pepper
spinach

water chestnuts
beans or peas, sprouted
pea pods
sliced black olives
toasted sesame seeds

VEGETABLE CHOP SUEY

1/4 cup sesame oil
1 1/2 cup shredded cabbage
1/2 cup sliced celery
1/2 cup sprouted peas
OR 1 pkg. frozen pea pods
1 cup bean sprouts
2-3 tbs. Bragg's liquid aminos
3/4 cup chicken bouillon
1 tbs. arrowroot
1/4 cup toasted slivered almonds
1 red pepper, cut in 2" strips

Heat oil in wok and add vegetables. Fry 2-3 minutes over
medium heat, stirring frequently. Add liquid aminos and 1/4
cup bouillon. Cover and simmer 4 minutes. Mix arrowroot
with remaining 1/2 cup bouillon and stir into vegetables.
Cook 2 minutes or until sauce thickens. Serve over rice.
Top with almonds.

IMITATION CRAB, 'CREAMED' OVER RICE

2 tbs. butter, melted over low heat
2 tbs. rice flour, add over low heat
1 cup soy milk or goats milk, stirring to prevent lumping
Add Bragg's liquid aminos, pepper and Washters Sea and Land
seasoning to taste. Stir until thickened. Add 1/2 green
pepper, chopped and 1/3 cup chopped fresh parsley and cook
for 5 minutes.

Add 1/2-1 lb. imitation crab flakes and cook for 2-3 minutes.
Serve over brown rice or some other grain.

'CRABBY' VEGETABLES

1/4 cup butter, melt over low heat
2 green onions, chopped and 2 minced garlic buds, add and
saute. Add 10 oz. frozen or fresh vegetables, a few shakes
of pepper and 1/2 lb. imitation crab flakes. Cover and steam
for 10 minutes.

Add at the end 2 tbs. fresh lemon and serve with brown rice,
amaranth or millet. Can also be served over Japanese
buckwheat noodles or rice noodles.

CAULIFLOWER CASSEROLE

1 medium cauliflower
3 tbs. butter
3 tbs. rice flour
1 1/2 cup soy milk or goat's milk
1/2-tsp. salt or Bragg's liquid aminos
1/8 tsp. pepper
1/2 cup fresh parsley (chopped) or 1 tsp. parsley flakes
    (optional)
3 hard-cooked eggs (thinly sliced)
1/2 cup crushed corn flakes or tortilla chips OR brown rice,
    crispy cereal OR crushed
2 tbs. melted butter

Separate washed cauliflower into flowerettes and steam for a
few minutes. It should still be quite firm.

Meanwhile, melt 3 tbs. butter in saucepan. Stir in rice
flour; add soy milk and cook, stirring constantly, until
thickened. Remove from heat and stir in seasoning and
parsley.

Layer cauliflower, sliced eggs and sauce into a greased
casserole. Toss crumbs with melted butter. Sprinkle over.

Bake, covered, in moderate oven (350) 25 minutes.   4-6
servings.

GOURMET SNAP BEANS

2 lbs. fresh green beans
1 tbs. sea salt
2 qts. boiling water
3 tbs. butter
2 tsp. lemon juice
2 tbs. minced fresh parsley
1/2 tsp. salt, or to taste
1/8 tsp. pepper, or to taste

Snap or cut off ends of beans. Just before cooking, wash
quickly under warm water. Add beans and 1 tbs. sea salt to
water. Bring quickly to boil and cook, uncovered, until
tender crisp (10-15 minutes), depending on the age of the
bean. Try one to test.

Drain beans into colander. To serve, immediately melt butter
in large skillet. Add drained beans and stir until hot.
Remove from heat; add lemon juice, parsley and seasoning.
Stir.

SPRINGTIME SPINACH

1 lb. fresh spinach, washed
1/2 - 1 tsp. salt (sprinkled on spinach)
1/4 cup butter
1 cup diced or shredded beets
2 tbs. lemon juice
1/2 tsp. salt
1/8 tsp. pepper
1 tbs. chopped fresh parsley (optional)
2-4 hard cooked eggs (yolks and whites divided)

Sprinkle spinach with salt and cook in water that clings to
leaves in heavy saucepan, covered, for 10 minutes. Drain and
chop coarsely. Heat butter in skillet; add beets and heat
thoroughly (If raw beets are used, cook for 20 minutes in
skillet with 1 tbs. oil, covered, before adding butter.) Add
rest of ingredients except egg yolks. Mash yolks and
sprinkle on top. (Makes 4-5 servings)

STEAMED VEGETABLES

1 1/2 to 2 pounds mixed vegetables (cauliflower florets,
   broccoli florets, sliced carrot, zucchini and yellow
   squash)
1/2 cup butter
3 cloves garlic, minced
2 tablespoons chopped parsley
1/4 teaspoon oregano (optional)
Salt, pepper

Place vegetables on rack in steamer and steam over boiling
water until tender-crisp, about 15 minutes or less.
Meanwhile, heat butter, add garlic and parsley and saute
lightly. Stir in oregano and season to taste with salt and
pepper. Pour some of butter mixture over each serving of
vegetables. Makes 6 to 8 servings.

PANACHE OF POTATOES A LA DUCHESSE

3 medium russet potatoes
3 medium yams
2 egg yolks
1/4 cup butter, melted
Dash nutmeg
Salt, pepper

Peel and quarter potatoes and yams. Cook potatoes in boiling
water 10 minutes or until done. Cook yams in boiling water
about 25 minutes or until done. Drain thoroughly and allow
to dry slightly. Put potatoes and yams through ricer and
blend well. Beat in egg yolks, butter and nutmeg. Season to

taste with salt and pepper. Using pastry bag fitted with large fluted tube, pipe swirls of mixture around entree on serving platter. Makes 10 to 12 servings.

Note: If preferred, recipe may be served in casserole. To obtain same number of servings, double amount of recipe and place in casserole. Bake at 350 degrees 10 to 5 minutes to heat through.

KABOCHA PUMPKIN SOUP

2 onions (chopped)
4 cloves garlic (chopped)

Saute in toasted sesame oil or corn oil until translucent - in soup kettle.

Fill kettle with water to 2/3 full. Add 2 small or large kabocha pumpkin* (skin and all) - steamed and chunked. (*Also known as "Japanese" pumpkin at Ralph's - grayish in color.)

Add a Burdock Root (size of large carrot) - sliced (also called "Gobo"). Add 2 strips Kombu (soaked 10 minutes) and cut in 1/2" pieces.

Add: 1 small daikon (white Japanese radish) - chopped, 1 stalk celery - chopped, 1 parsnip - chopped

Simmer 1 1/2 hours until smooth. Possible optional seasonings: parsley, parch "baking blend" or pumpkin spice, OR put in bowl and add Miso Master white.

IMITATION CRAB-VEGETABLE SOUP

9 cups chicken broth, imitation chicken broth, OR instant
    broth mix (yeast-free)
1 lb. imitation crab flakes
1 small head nappa cabbage (cut up)
1 zucchini (large) or 2 small - sliced in thin rounds
Salt or Bragg's liquid aminos - to taste
White pepper - a few shakes
Sesame oil - a few drops
2 green onions - chopped (reserve some green top pieces for
    garnish)

Heat all ingredients to boiling. If desired, add few drops of sesame oil. Sprinkle with green onion tops or chives for garnish.

BUTTERY GRATED CARROTS

2 lbs. carrots
1 tbs. oil
1/4 tsp. finely chopped garlic
1/2 tsp. salt
1/8 tsp. pepper
1/4 cup butter

Pare or scrub carrots; grate or shred into large skillet with
tight fitting cover. Toss with oil, garlic, salt and pepper,
and 2 tbs. water. Cook, covered, over medium heat, stirring
occasionally, 10-12 minutes, or until tender. Remove from
heat. Toss with butter to coat. (Serves 4-6)

BUTTERY GRATED BEETS

Use 2 lbs. beets instead of carrots. Proceed as above, but
cook beets 20 minutes or until tender. Remove from heat.
Toss lightly with butter and 1-2 tbs. lemon juice (adjust to
taste). (4-6 servings)

BUTTERY GRATED TURNIPS

Use 3 lbs. white turnips instead of carrots. Proceed as
above, but cook turnips 15 minutes or until tender. Then to
evaporate liquid, cook, uncovered, over very low heat for 5
minutes. Remove from heat. Toss with butter, 1-2 tbs. lemon
juice, 1/4 cup chopped parsley - until turnips are coated.
(4-6 servings)

LEMON BROCCOLI

2 to 2 1/2 pounds broccoli
2 cloves garlic, halved
2 tbs. oil
Juice of 1/2 lemon
Salt, pepper
Lemon slices

Split thick broccoli stems to heads and steam over boiling
water until barely tender. Drain and cut into large pieces.

Saute garlic in oil just until garlic begins to brown.
Discard garlic and add broccoli to seasoned oil. Cook until
tender, turning pieces frequently. Sprinkle with lemon
juice. Season to taste with salt and pepper. Serve with
lemon slices. Makes 8 servings.

MILLET VEGETABLE SOUP

2 onions finely chopped
1/4 cabbage head, finely chopped
6-7 cups of water
1 cup millet
2 diced carrots
Sea salt
1 bay leaf
Pinch of thyme
1 tbs. of Miso Master White (paste)
Finely chopped cilantro

Roast the millet and put in boiling water with all the
vegetables, except the last three ingredients. Lower the
fire to simmer, for 30 minutes. Keep pot covered while
cooking. When ready, include last three ingredients,
dissolving the Miso in some of the soup. If you fee you need
more mso, feel free to add more to your taste. Serve hot or
cold.

BEAN SOUP

1 cup navy beans
1-2 strips komb or wakame
2-3 large leeks
1 onion
2-3 bay leaves (optional)
1 teaspoon oil
White or light miso to taste (or sea salt)
Fresh or dried herbs (basil or dill goes well with this dish)
1 carrot

Wash and soak navy beans 2-8 hours. Drain. Bring to a boil
in 4 cups water, with sea vegetable and bay leaves for one
hour, covered, or pressure cook 40 minutes. Beans should be
very soft.

Slice leeks in half lengthwise and wash very well to remove
all dirt; slice fine. Dice onion.

Saute onion and leek over medium heat until soft and clear -
10-15 minutes.

When the beans are soft, add to sauteed leeks. Add 2-3 cups
of water if needed for creamy consistency. Simmer 20-30
minutes over low heat. Puree part of the beans to make
smooth soup.

Chop fresh herbs (basil or dill) and add with miso and/or
salt. Blanch carrot matchsticks for garnish.

AVOCADO DRESSING

2 tbs. oil
1 large ripe avocado
3 tbs. lemon juice
1/4 - 1/2 tsp. salt (to taste)
Dash pepper
Dash cayenne
Optional: Dash garlic powder

Mash avocado with fork; shake all ingredients together in a jar, or put everything into a blender or food processor and blend until quite smooth. (Makes 1 cup)

SESAME SALAD DRESSING

1/2 cup vegetable oil (unrefined)
1/4 cup toasted sesame seeds
2 tbsp. fresh lemon juice
1/2 tsp. sea salt
Optional: 1 cup chopped parsley

Blend in blender until nearly smooth. Refrigerate.

Other dressings are made by CARDINI and are free of vinegar - Caesar Dressing & Lemon Herb Dressing.

FRESH HERB BUTTER

1 green onion OR 1/2 of small onion AND/OR 2 cloves garlic
    (chopped)
1/4 cup packed tarragon, basil, parsley OR cilantro leaves
1/4 tsp. salt
1 tsp. lemon juice
1/4 tsp. white pepper
Dash cayenne
1/2 cup unsalted butter, softened

With food processor running, drop onion and/or garlic in and process until minced. Add herbs and salt and process until chopped (20 seconds). Add rest of ingredients and process until well mixed. Use as is, or transfer to wax paper or plastic wrap; roll into cylinder about 1" thick or 8" long. Freeze until ready to use. Makes 1/2 cup.

TOMATOE BUTTER

1 green onion OR 1/2 small brown onion AND/OR 2 cloves garlic
1/4 tsp. salt
1 1/2 tbs. fresh tomatoes
1 tsp. lemon juice
1/4 tsp. white pepper
Dash cayenne
1/2 cup unsalted butter, softened
Process as in recipe above. Use immediately or freeze.
Makes 1/2 cup.

LEMON-SESAME SAUCE
(For asparagus or broccoli)

1/4 cup butter
Juice of 1/2 lemon
1 tbs. toasted sesame seeds
10 drops liquid sweetener OR dash of barley malt powder
1/4 tsp. garlic salt
Optional: A little grated lemon peel

Melt butter and add lemon juice and peel, if desired, sesame
seeds and garlic salt. Stir and heat. Remove from heat and
add sweetener.

ORDERFORM

Please send the book

" CANDIDA. THE EPIDEMIC OF THIS CENTURY: SOLVED "

Unit Price : $10
Postage : $2.50

California Residents. add 6% Sales tax : 60cts

NAME :
STREET :
CITY :   STATE :   ZIP :

Please forward to : LDS Publications
4318 Beaucroft Ct
Westlake Village. Ca 91361